BECOMING AND BEING A PHYSICIAN

Structured around personal stories, this book provides a rigorous review of current thinking and research on the physician's life cycle. The book considers the trajectories and factors that influence a doctor's development over decades of a medical career.

Taking an integrated approach, the authors consider the formal stages of a physician's training including medical school, residency training, and practice, and review discourses around professionalism, competency-based education, lifelong learning, expertise development, reflection, and narrative that merge into the construct of medical professional identity formation.

Reflecting the dramatic changes that have occurred in the physician's role, job description, and reality of modern clinical practice, further compounded by the pandemic, this new book will support and encourage medical educators to ensure that the enduring values of the medical profession prevail.

Becoming and Being a Physician

A Developmental Journey

Shmuel P. Reis
Adina L. Kalet
W. Wayne Weston

CRC Press
Taylor & Francis Group
Boca Raton London New York

CRC Press is an imprint of the
Taylor & Francis Group, an **informa** business

Cover design: Kristina Grosbart

Line editing: Lahevet Pollack

First edition published 2025
by CRC Press
2385 NW Executive Center Drive, Suite 320, Boca Raton, FL 33431

and by CRC Press
4 Park Square, Milton Park, Abingdon, Oxon, OX14 4RN

CRC Press is an imprint of Taylor & Francis Group, LLC

© 2025 Shmuel P. Reis, Adina L. Kalet, and W. Wayne Weston

ISBN: 9781032830551 (hbk)
ISBN: 9781032830568 (pbk)
ISBN: 9781003507529 (ebk)

DOI: 10.1201/9781003507529

Typeset in Sabon
by Deanta Global Publishing Services, Chennai, India

Contents

Preface

One night I was called to see a patient who had died. He and his family had been in my care for the last 40 years. Deteriorating slowly over a few years, he had signed his advance directive, rejected interventions, and had a smooth transition to comfort care. I had visited him a few days prior; he was already unconscious and peaceful. After completing the death certificate paperwork, I sat in the living room with his wife and two of his siblings. We reminisced about how we had first met, and about salient moments en route. One of them said, "You can retire now. You've taken good care of us for the last 40 years and supported Dad in dying peacefully at home, thank you."

This book is a labor of love. Ten years of writing, longer in the thinking, provide the broader context for the long journey and deeply intimate moments I shared with this family. I was almost overcome with emotions as we finalized this manuscript. This brainchild, the fruit of more than five decades of reflection on becoming and being a physician, is about to be born. This journey has been a mixture of wonder, joy, self-doubt, and downright distress. Medicine has turned out to be the most wonderful vocation for me, yet at times it has been horrible. Nevertheless, I would not choose another path if reincarnated. A sense of fulfillment prevails; I feel only great fortune and deep gratitude for this privilege.

The idea behind this book was conceived while I was doing my Master of Health Professions Education (MHPE) in Maastricht, the Netherlands, just before the turn of the century. I was fascinated by the insight that developing as a clinician was not incremental but happened in discrete nodal points where a qualitative threshold was crossed and, as a result, the clinician's comfort zone was enlarged (more about this in the book). I planned on interviewing exemplars about the experience of breakthroughs and had a few narratives collected from colleagues in North America. However, the project was washed away by the tide of intensive life and subsequently transformed into the idea of writing this book. I met Wayne once in the early 1990s when I participated in a medical education class he facilitated and remained in communication with him. Once the idea of the book matured, I knew he was the ideal partner. Later, we both felt that we were missing a feminine perspective in our inquiry and approached Adina. We were aware of her unique contributions to medical education and were very glad she was interested. The rest is history.

I wasn't one of those people who knew they would become a physician at an early age. My late mother, blessed be her soul, used to tell me that I could become whatever I wanted to be except a physician, since I tended to turn pale at the sight of blood. This changed when I was in my first battle as a soldier in June 1967. Aged 19, I was assigned to carry the dead and wounded on a stretcher to the doctor's station. It struck me that the doctor, going about his work surrounded by a few medics, was an island of sanity in the sea of madness. At that moment, medicine became an option.

At the age of 23, newly married, I started studying in Paris, France. My wife gave birth to our eldest daughter that first year, with me sitting beside her bed studying for an exam, a scene repeated three years later with our son's birth. In the summer of 1973, we moved back to Israel straight into the Yom Kippur War, and I was mobilized into military service. Although school started in January of 1974, I was only able to finally join my class in late February. While serving, I studied from colleagues' notes and the *Robbins Basic Pathology* textbook. A few flashes of memory from medical school: a superb small group, a case-based biochemistry class (bilirubin metabolism) facilitated by Professor Hershko, a physician–scientist destined to win a Nobel Prize three decades later. I recall in intimate detail the stories the late Rosalie Ber, our clinical skills instructor, told of the devotion of her late husband, a physician, to his patients. I still feel the deep emotion I felt when many years later when I replaced her, that beloved teacher, recently deceased, in running the medical education unit of my alma mater.

While in medical school, I worked as a nurse. Once, I accidentally administered an overdose of morphine to a kidney transplant patient. Luckily, no permanent harm was done. In the summer of my fifth year of medical school, I shadowed a rural family physician for a few weeks, an experience which solidified my decision to follow that path. On my first night on call as an intern in the emergency room, I was caring for a

French-speaking diabetic woman with chest pain. After confirming her ECG and labs were normal, I discharged her. Early the next morning, she returned with florid pulmonary edema and died—I had misjudged the seriousness of her situation. In her anguish, she called to me, "Mon jeune docteur, aidez-moi" (*My young doctor, help me*). With no debriefing or discussion afterward, I was left alone to process my fatal misjudgment. Other than this tragedy, and perhaps because of it, my internship year was a peak learning experience. I delivered 50 babies, saw lice on a patient's head for the first time, and conducted my first thorough literature search in the library.

In May 1978, I started my residency. One morning, during my year-long internal medicine rotation, I presented a puzzling patient case to the chief of our service. He utterly astounded me by responding, "Familial nephrogenic diabetes insipidus presented as gout—four cases described in the *NEJM*..." This was well before PubMed enabled digital searching of literature. This man just knew everything instantly! I acquired skills, gained confidence, and developed habits of mind. In my spare time, I started practicing medicine in the village where I lived, also serving the two adjacent tiny rural communities. While on my obstetrics and gynecology clerkship, I advocated for a patient who, as a child, had undergone cardiac surgery to correct a very complicated congenital abnormality, tetralogy of Fallot. She now needed the best possible care for her high-risk pregnancy. Years later, she asked me to contribute a chapter to a book compiling narratives she had written during and after this period. This was my introduction (among others) to narrative medicine.

Subsequently, I started my first family medicine rotation with my mentor, the late Tomi Spenser, to whom I dedicate this book. We visited one large Arab village clinic daily and each of three to four small communities twice a week. Tomi taught me many clinical skills, including IUD insertion and minor surgery, but he also schooled me in medical recordkeeping (POMR [Problem-Oriented Medical Record]), research in practice, home visits, a family orientation, and more. We frequently met in his living room, where he and his wife (also a GP) nurtured me with food, teaching, and affection.

In June 1982, I was mobilized for service in the First Lebanon War. This was a brutal introduction to battlefield doctoring. I needed to tend to casualties among the soldiers in my unit as well as local civilians, sometimes under fire. During this early part of my career journey, I was involved in building a rural health center that finally opened in February 1984. This involved many firsts, such as learning to plan, lobbying the government, establishing hospice-at-home and hospital-at-home programs. I learned almost everything on the job. Throughout this time, I remained active nationally with my professional organizations and took on leadership roles in the Israel Association of Family Physicians.

Visiting departments of family medicine and participating in conferences opened my eyes to new ways of doing things. In 1989, the Israel Association of Family Physicians hosted the World Organization of Family Doctors (WONCA) World Conference in Jerusalem. Our practice thrived, as did our ability to be innovative in broadening the scope of practice, educating excellent residents, and conducting research. We were pioneers in introducing an electronic medical record into our family medicine practice with the support of a generous gift from a person I revived by CPR at Ben Gurion Airport in February 1990 as I was on my way to North America for a monthlong sabbatical—the trip where I first met Wayne.

My first marriage ended in divorce. I had been an absent father to my four children. I strived to make amends for this in my second marriage.

My father became ill in his early 70s. When he passed away in 1991, I was at his bedside at home. During those years, my identity as a family practitioner evolved away from the ideal of being the best family doctor I could be on my own toward the realization that without a strong community and involvement in teaching, my aims would not be achieved. I was rapidly developing professional and academic skills while also becoming a medico–politician. In 1992, I became Chairman of Family Medicine at the Rappaport Faculty of Medicine at the Technion, Israel, which consolidated my new identity as the academic–practitioner I am to this day. Deeply involved with the national and international academic family medicine scene, I attended many conferences, traveled widely, and forged many professional collaborations. I was drawn to honing my expertise as an educator. Completing the MHPE in Maastricht was a transformative experience, as it inspired both deep learning and a painful realization that I had been ignorant of this scholarly discipline. One consequence was a yearlong sabbatical (2007–2008), which transformed me from one immersed in academic family medicine to my new identity as a medical education scholar. In the second decade of this century, I was part of the team that established a new medical school in the Galilee and continued many projects with my international colleagues.

When I reached retirement age in Israel (67), my first grandchild was born, I was recruited to head the Center for Medical Education at the Hebrew University of Jerusalem Faculty of Medicine, and I left my 38-year career in health center-based clinical work, maintaining only a small local practice. I was becoming grandfatherly in all aspects of my life.

The last three years, while less hectic, have been challenging in new and different ways. Most central to my identity is my role as co-chair of the *Lancet* Commission on medicine, Nazism, and the Holocaust, which has led to intensive international collaboration, a great deal of remote teaching around the globe, and writing for publication.

Writing this book has allowed me to deeply reflect on the past 53 years of becoming and being a physician. In reviewing my own journey to this point, I have emphasized the positive and spared you the most painful low moments—the many errors, failures, quarrels, and relationship ruptures. Both positive and painful experiences have played their roles in my own becoming. I hope this book facilitates your own reflections and invites you to join the conversation. I look forward to hearing from you.

—*Shmuel P. Reis*

How did I become the physician–educator I am today? Let me start at the beginning.

My mother was a Holocaust survivor. Celia Kalmanowitz arrived in the United States as a 14-year-old refugee from a displaced persons camp in US-occupied Germany. I was born eight years later. Holiday meals with my family of survivors were a literal Tower of Babel in Yiddish, Polish, Russian, and English (for the children). Harrowing stories and partisan anthems mingled with the gossip of the day.

These people modeled resilience in the face of unbearable trauma and loss. They demonstrated how to rebuild dignity and community even as geopolitical catastrophes echoed across the generations, impacting each individual's mental and physical health in distinctive ways. After a feast, it was not rare for one of my relatives to end the evening in the bedroom on supplemental oxygen and intravenous diuretics.

Very young, I learned that while strong character skills are important, one's survival might depend on having a good doctor available.

As a child, I struggled with what is now called a learning disability. I didn't read until my very attentive fourth-grade teacher, Mr. James Garnets, raised the bar by suggesting to my mother that I might be smart. She took it from there. Every day that summer, my mother and I walked to the public library. We read every book on the young readers shelf, and she had me write a short report on each of them. By the next school year, to everyone's delight, I was reading above my grade level.

As a teenager, I dreamed of being a dancer. When it became clear I was not good enough to make it as a performer, I turned to teaching dance. That was when the lightbulb went on. Guiding others was miraculous, fun, and satisfying.

So, how did I end up in medicine when there were other, easier paths to becoming an educator? It was the early 1970s, and opportunities for women were rapidly expanding. I knew I had more choices than those who had come before me, and I pushed myself to make the most of these opportunities. I hoped to build on the lessons learned from my family. But these vague notions and ambitions did not add up to an identity. I knew almost nothing about being a physician.

When the time arrived to look at colleges, my mother handed me an application to a new, innovative, accelerated six-year baccalaureate/MD program where students could become physicians without tackling "weed-out" college courses such as calculus and organic chemistry. There was no need to excel on the Medical College Admissions Test. Even though avoiding the competition was attractive, I was reluctant. After I was accepted, I struggled with whether to continue on this path. I was not certain I wanted to be a doctor but could think of no way to know for certain other than to try.

So, when I was 18, I signed a legally binding State of New York contract promising to work in an underserved urban community as a primary care physician in exchange for a nearly free medical education at the Sophie Davis School of Biomedical Education at the City College of New York (now the CUNY School of Medicine).

I loved the school and its mission. My exacting and inspiring mentors challenged me. Still, I fretted about losing myself. I promised to work hard to remain *me*. While many of my peers' trajectories were linear and predetermined—medical school to residency to fellowship to practice—my path was not clear. I took risks. I joined the first cohort of a brand-new residency program, a choice that placed me at the Bellevue Hospital Center in New York City during the earliest, most devastating years of the human immunodeficiency virus (HIV) epidemic.

Every physician has their own story of the challenges that tested their mettle and forged them into someone who runs toward—rather than away from—emergencies. My rite of passage occurred during my residency, working at the epicenter of the mysterious, terrifying, and fascinating epidemic that attacked and killed young adults while viciously ostracizing them from society. People and moments from those years are seared into my memory. Almost ten years after entering training, these experiences marked when I truly became a physician.

After residency, my new husband, Mark, and I convinced a foundation to fund us to visit and study innovative community-oriented medical schools in Israel and the Netherlands. As we traveled, our eyes opened to new avenues for our budding careers. We discovered that practicing clinical medicine was not the only way to "heal the world."

Educating physicians was intriguing. As a fellow in the then brand-new field of health services research, I learned the "hows and whys" and accumulated more role models and mentors. Rather than working at prestigious institutions, Mark and I returned to New York and practiced in a public community-based urban clinic. After all, that is what I had promised to do.

The decade I spent in primary care medicine at the Gouverneur Health Diagnostic and Treatment Center on the Lower East Side of Manhattan was the most creative of my life. The majority of my patients were non-English-speaking immigrants and refugees. In a clinic that struggled to attract and retain healthcare workers, our programs lured enthusiastic, well-trained physicians. Our center became a popular site for student and resident education, and our pipeline welcomed caring and excellent practitioners committed to working in medically under-served communities. This was difficult work. In addition to nurturing our own doctoring skills in an environment with severe resource restrictions, we had to be fundraisers, advocates, administrators, researchers, and expert communicators.

I pride myself on being a devoted mentor and colleague. While I would never have predicted this—and it took years of determination to develop the skills—I am now a successful grant-getter, researcher, writer, and lecturer. Recently, when preparing a speech for a national award, I understood that I was being recognized, fundamentally, for being persistent and dogged; dogged in collaborating with talented people who share a passion for educating physicians.

Of course, life happened along the way. At the same time as I was developing my chops as a physician and researcher, I became a wife, mother, daughter, sister, cousin, friend, and patient. I learned to juggle, balance, and integrate my family, friends, and work. I made sacrifices and mistakes. I spent time going up a few blind alleys and had my doubts. I lived my life in a series of careers rather than trying to do everything simultaneously.

The path has also been rocky. It turns out that a meaningful, purpose-filled career is not always the safest way to make a living. When political winds shift, people engaged in doing good work can lose funding, a heart-wrenching experience I have faced more than once. While loss is followed by anger, grief, and intense self-criticism, these moments have also been times when I discovered what and who really matter. It has been a privilege to discover who my friends are and who I might yet become in the process.

Beginning with my mother and then Mr. Garnets in fourth grade, my mentors have seen, believed in, and challenged me to do more and be better while doing good. To my many mentors, those still alive and those who are no longer with us (including Mildred Gordon, PhD; Pyser Edelsack, MSW; and Jo Anne Earp, ScD), I say: *thank you, thank you, thank you.* Because of the circumstances of her life, my mother, a fierce and compassionate protector of her family and her people, didn't get to fully realize her potential. She died unexpectedly the year before I had my first child. I try every day to honor and celebrate her.

Parenting taught me to say yes as much as possible and no only when necessary. That is how I became entangled in this love letter to our profession, *Becoming and Being a Physician*, with thought partners and fellow travelers, Drs. Shmuel Reis and Wayne Weston. I am grateful for this partnership.

A mentor once pointed out that we will have only one career in retrospect. Of course, he was right; we can never know how it will unfold. We can only try to make good choices, tend to our relationships, take risks whenever we can, try not to be too fragile, and respect our losses.

I have many joys in my life. I draw, paint, and garden even if I never became a dancer or learned calculus. I still love the journey. I believe my mother would have been proud.

—*Adina L. Kalet*

In some cases, an illness can change the shape of the rest of your life. In my case, it was having appendicitis at age nine. Because my appendix had ruptured, I was seriously ill with peritonitis and then suffered two episodes of bowel obstruction requiring surgery—three operations within a month. I made a remarkably quick recovery and was soon back at school. My mother was so grateful for the good medical care that had saved her son that she frequently commented on the importance of doctors and made it clear to me that being a doctor would be a wonderful goal. It wasn't long before I decided that I would aim for a life in medicine and never considered anything else. My understanding of what this meant was naive and simplistic. No one in my family had ever gone to university or pursued a professional career, so I had no role model to guide me. I sometimes wonder if this early choice of a career sidetracked some of the other tasks of identity formation.

I was always very shy and avoided situations where I might be embarrassed. In high school, I joined the Camera Club and soon became its president, which resulted in my being asked to be the editor of the school yearbook. When I had a role to play, I felt less nervous and became more confident.

When it was time to apply to university, I naively applied only to the University of Toronto Medical School so that I could live at home and keep costs down. But continuing to live at home removed the challenges associated with independence. At that time, the Toronto program consisted of a two-year premed curriculum followed by a four-year conventional medical curriculum. Premed courses included philosophy, English, anthropology, psychology, zoology, chemistry, and physics.

I felt challenged by medical school and focused on learning the prescribed curriculum. I got good marks but became more introverted and boring. I had a summer job in a nursing home one year and, in another year, worked at a huge provincial "lunatic asylum" where people with presumed mental illness were housed, but without sufficient staff to treat them—conditions best described by Charles Dickens. Both experiences during medical school sensitized me to the need for better care for people struggling with mental illness. I started reading books about Freud and his theories, as well as Erik Erikson's stages of development. This helped me realize that students' readiness or ability to learn certain concepts or skills depends on their stage of development.

In my final year, I met and fell in love with the woman who would become my wife and the mother of our five children. She continues to show me how to love and care for others.

After a one-year rotating internship, all in the hospital, I was licensed to practice in 1965. Longer training in general practice was not yet available. During my urology rotation, the senior resident told me about a small-town practice seeking an additional physician. It was in his hometown of Tavistock, Ontario. My fiancé and I went for an interview to meet with the physicians and liked what we saw. After completing my rotating internship, we were married, enjoyed a brief honeymoon, and moved from Toronto to Tavistock—population 1,300—a lot of changes to adjust to all at once. I was too young, only 25! Some of my patients commented, "Are you sure you're a doctor?"

I had focused all my attention on doing well in school and had not had to struggle with my personal development. Perhaps that stimulated my interest in how we mature. I started reading about how others had coped with medical training. Doctor X had just published *Intern*, in which he journaled his thoughts and feelings about his experiences.

I quickly realized that I was educated to manage common medical conditions in the hospital but was unfamiliar with many conditions presenting in the community, especially mental illness, skin problems, and musculoskeletal conditions. I remember my excitement at discovering Ian McWhinney's first book, *The Early Signs of Illness*, published in 1964, the year I finished medical school. Finally, a book written by a GP, describing common conditions not mentioned in the usual medical texts.

For ten years I practiced comprehensive family medicine, including an office practice in Tavistock, house calls, care of patients in the hospital and in the emergency department in Stratford, Ontario, full obstetric care, and teaching medical students during their one-month clinical clerkship. Our practice provided care in emergencies 24 hours a day, every day of the year. I still remember some of the patients I cared for almost 60 years ago. I enjoyed helping medical students begin to understand that there is more to healthcare than diagnosis and treatment. After five years in Tavistock, I was invited to fill a recently vacated seven-month academic position at the University of Western Ontario (now Western University). My partners in Tavistock agreed to let me go. At the end of the locum, I did not feel ready and returned to Tavistock—there was so much more to learn about caring for patients. Five years later, I received another invitation to join an academic practice associated with the Department of Family Medicine at Western. I was flattered by the offer and accepted.

Soon after moving to Western, I joined a small group in the Department of Family Medicine studying patient–clinician communication and the patient-centered clinical method. This led to ongoing collaboration with the group and the publication of a textbook on this topic, now in its fourth edition.[1]

I had the privilege of working under the guidance of Ian McWhinney for 20 years. Recognizing the importance of scholarship, he established a graduate program in 1977 and a special research center in 1978, attracting family physicians and other clinicians from around the world. He recognized my interest in medical education and asked me to create a course, which would become one of the main courses of the Graduate Studies Program in Family Medicine at Western. I taught Teaching and Learning in the Health Sciences over the next 30 years before passing it on to five of the program's graduates. That became my passion over the rest of my career. Recognizing my ignorance of teaching and education, I enlisted the help of some of the best teachers at Western, McMaster University, and the University of Toronto.

---

1   Stewart, M., Brown, J. B., Weston, W. W., Freeman, T., Ryan, B. L., McWilliam, C. L., & McWhinney, I. R. (2024). *Patient-centered medicine: Transforming the clinical method* (4th ed.). CRC Press.

During a visit to Western, Shmuel sat in on a session of the teaching and learning course, and we learned that we shared an interest in models of the personal development of physicians. He contacted me about ten years ago, and we began sending our ideas back and forth. I scoured bookstores for books on anything related to teaching and learning, as well as personal stories of students' experiences during medical training, and developed a huge personal library. I enjoyed sharing what I had learned with others and learning from them. The graduate program's multinational reach led to invitations to consult with other programs across Canada and the United States, Scotland, New Zealand, the United Arab Emirates, and Kazakhstan, with a variety of requests to support the development and teaching of problem-based learning, faculty development, curricular change, and leadership development.

I retired from practice in 2004 after 39 years of patient care, but continue to enjoy my involvement in academic activities. Many people have supported me in my academic journey, especially Ian McWhinney, who was a powerful example and guide. I have always had a hard time expressing my feelings and am learning that this may come across as indifference and interfere with communication. My wife has shown me a much better way and didn't give up on me when I lost my way.

—*W. Wayne Weston*

Acknowledgments

The creation of this book would not have been possible without the support and help of a few consultants, friends, and professionals: Prof. Jeff Borkan, MD, PhD, who suggested this book's title and rooted for us; Prof. Carol Herbert, CM, MD, DSc, CCFP, FCFP, FCAHS, FRACGP (Hon), who reviewed our discussion of the different developmental stages and pointed out to us that we should greatly increase our focus on the development of female physicians; Prof. Yvonne Steinert, PhD, who commended us on thorough referencing alongside additional feedback; and Prof. Eric Marcus, MD, for his inspiration and generosity in permitting our use of his "Wild Strawberries" piece.

Rita Charon, MD, PhD, and Ron Epstein, MD, FAAHPM, who generously provided the Prologue and Epilogue.

Lahevet Pollack, our language editor, the embodiment of professionalism and editing from the heart; and Simona Shahaf, Shmuel's administrative assistant, who joined relatively late in the journey and made a big difference.

Finally, our CRC Press/Taylor & Francis editor, Jo Koster, whom we met almost by accident, and who encouraged and supported us all the way up to the completion of this work.

Authors

Shmuel P. Reis, MD, MHPE, is a family physician in northern Israel in his 47th year of practice. He is a faculty member at the Holon Institute of Technology, where he teaches courses such as The Doctor in the Digital Age and Patient–Doctor Discourse in the Digital Age at the institute's new BSc in Digital Medical Technologies program. He is the former academic head of the Center for Medical Education at the Hebrew University of Jerusalem Faculty of Medicine, and the former head of the School for Competencies Education in Residency of the Israeli Medical Association Scientific Council (Israel's equivalent of the ACGME). He is also the founder and past chair of the Israeli Society for Medical Education (HEALER). He is co-chair of the *Lancet* Commission on medicine, Nazism, and the Holocaust (MNH) and course director for Israeli faculty development of MNH teachers, as well as for both Hebrew and English MNH massive open online courses (MOOCs). His major research and education foci are medicine, Nazism, and the Holocaust, patient–doctor–computer communication, and the physician life cycle. He can be reached at: shmuelre@hit.ac.il.

Adina L. Kalet, MD, MPH, a general internist, is Professor of Medicine and Medical Education at the Medical College of Wisconsin, and previously Professor of Medicine and Surgery at the New York University Grossman School of Medicine. She teaches, mentors, and has led several cross-disciplinary groups of educators and researchers working to link education and health services research methodology to study the connection between medical education and long-term outcomes in learners and patients. She writes and speaks regularly on transforming medical education, clinical skills and professionalism remediation, educational technology, mentoring, and professional identity formation assessment. She co-directs the US site of the University of Maastricht's Master of Health Professions Education (MHPE) program and leads several annual mentor development programs. In 2023, along with Dr. Calvin L. Chou, she published the second edition of *Remediation in Medical Education: A Mid-Course Correction* and received two national career awards—the National Board of Medical Examiners (NBME) John P. Hubbard Award and the Association of Academic Medical Colleges (AAMC) Award for Excellence in Medical Education. She has served on, and now chairs, the International Academic Review Committee (IARC), providing counsel to the Ben-Gurion University of the Negev School of Medicine in Israel.

W. Wayne Weston, MD, CCFP, FCFP, is Emeritus Professor of Family Medicine at the Schulich School of Medicine and Dentistry at Western University in Ontario, Canada. He taught a graduate-level course on teaching and learning in the health sciences for 30 years, attracting students from around the world. He has published 200 articles and book chapters in various journals and is co-author of two books on patient-centered medicine: *Patient-Centered Medicine: Transforming the Clinical Method*, 4th edition published in 2024; and *Challenges and Solutions in Patient-Centered Care: A Casebook*, published in 2002. He has offered over 500 presentations and workshops on many topics including patient-centered communication, problem-based learning, clinical teaching, professionalism, and dementia worldwide. He was a member of several national education committees, including chairing the advisory committee for the Institute for Healthcare Communication. He has received numerous awards for his work, including four national awards for teaching.

List of Figures

List of Tables

List of Abbreviations

ADDIE	Analyze, design, develop, implement, evaluate
AMA	American Medical Association
BMJ	*British Medical Journal*
CBME	Competency-based medical education
CHAT	Cultural–historical activity theory
CME	Continuous medical education
CPD	Continuous professional development
DEI	Diversity, equity, and inclusion
DIT	Defining Issues Test
DKA	Diabetic ketoacidosis
DLC	Doctor's life cycle
DP	Deliberate practice
ECG	Electrocardiogram
EMR	Electronic medical record
ER	Emergency room
FCM	Four Component Model
GMC	General Medical Council
GP	General practitioner, or general practice
HIV	Human immunodeficiency virus
ICU	Intensive care unit
IUD	Intrauterine device
JAMA	*Journal of the American Medical Association*
LGBTQIA+	Lesbian, gay, bisexual, transgender, queer, intersex, asexual, and additional identities
MAL	Master adaptive learner
MCW	Medical College of Wisconsin

MHPE	Master of Health Professions Education
MI	Myocardial infarction
NEJM	*New England Journal of Medicine*
NM	Narrative medicine
OSCE	Objective structured clinical examination
PGE	Postgraduate education
PIE	Professional identity essay
PIF	Professional identity formation
POMR	Problem-oriented medical record
PPD	Personal and professional development
PSSP	Personality and social structure perspective
UME	Undergraduate medical education
URiM	Underrepresented in medicine
ZPD	Zone of proximal development

Prologue

Rita Charon, MD, PhD
Professor of Medicine and Medical Humanities and Ethics
Columbia University
New York, New York

Don't read this book unless you are poised for transformation. While providing a comprehensive review of decades of academic research and scholarship on adult learning, *Becoming and Being a Physician* gifts its reader with moments of instantaneous clarity. The advanced clinical mentor observes as the junior resident fumbles in front of a patient terrified that she has developed the breast cancer that led to her mother's death. The mentor pays exquisite attention to the scene, describes it in detail in his notebook, and then reflects with the resident about the unanswerable questions that arise, resulting in deep learning for them both. The senior resident empties her hospital locker on the last day of her training, feeling in her body the crushing implications of the moment. An intern notices her clutching her chest, puts the scene together in an intuitive instant, and hands her a bottle of curative antacid. Instead of reaching for an illness script, the intern recognizes a moment suffused with meaning for a fellow traveler in the shared cosmos of their medical lives.

The three authors of this book give their readers an extraordinary resource. They've summarized frameworks for professional development from myriad disciplines and practices—the sociology of professions, business, dentistry, the ministry. They've taken seriously the ecology of professional development. Learning from a catholic range of viewpoints and transdisciplinary research traditions, they've integrated influential thinking about stages of adult learning as they pertain to physicians, giving us deeply informed foundations upon which to construct our future educational paths.

As always with great texts, the form holds the wisdom. The surfeit of structures described in these pages—stages, phases, theories, constructs, transitions, goals, accomplishments—seems to suggest an orderly, predictable process of professional development from medical novice to expert. And yet the text is saturated with questioning, uncertainty, yearning, and stories. By introducing each chapter with a narrative account, with most of the narratives shared by one of the co-authors, we readers know we are in the presence of *persons* with histories, memories, regrets, and epiphanies of their own. Shmuel's transatlantic management of his friend's acute leukemia, Wayne's sudden transition from doctor to cardiac patient, Adina's mentorship by Lew Goldfrank in the Bellevue ER to comprehend her radical love for an impossible patient—these co-authors don't hide behind their byline but take our hands, putting themselves on the line to model the depth of *self* needed to practice medicine.

These are not random recollections by three physicians as they exit their practice of medicine. Rather, the authors confront the challenges facing all medical educators responding to today's healthcare systems. They address the assessment of clinical expertise, the powers of mentorship, and the *phronesis*, or practical wisdom, of Aristotle. They probe moral development—including moral distress and injury—and the ethical discernment necessary to clarify physicians' duties in the face of injustice and abuse of power.

Considering students' moral and ethical development calls forth the affordances of narrative and reflective practices to help students grapple with the emotional and ontological toll of medical work. Telling stories, writing and reading narratives, dwelling on past experiences, and claiming what their dreams and memories reveal can expose students' inner lives to themselves. This self-awareness both deepens each student's grasp of their emerging professional identity and opens dialogue among students about the social and value ecologies of medical education.

Among the challenges faced by medical educators are remediating students whose clinical and personal skills are subpar and addressing the woundedness of students whose witnessing of patients' illnesses can summon traumas of their own. How, the authors ask, can we ably face and ultimately prevent the problems of addiction and suicide among our learners and colleagues? They devote two chapters to investigating racial injustice in healthcare as exacerbated by COVID-19, misogyny in medicine, and discrimination along sexual identity, ability, and cultural identity lines. Microaggressions, implicit and explicit bias, and harassment by faculty and trainees are addressed along with descriptions of diversity, equity, and inclusion (DEI) projects and upstander training to ally with those targeted by discrimination.

The book's penultimate chapter examines the capacity of professional identity formation to address the social, moral, and justice challenges facing medical education while preparing students for their professional lives of service. We readers gradually come to understand that the education being proposed is indeed transformative. Each student can face their own singular demons and inspirations. Each student can—with mentors and coaches committed to their journey—identify discomforts, doubts, and fears in a "zone of proximal development" where they need not retreat to their conventional comfort zone but can dare to move ahead toward as yet unexplored cognitive and affective terrain. Have we medical educators ourselves developed our formative strengths and ethical insights? Guiding students to learn of their professional identity values may encourage us to do the same within our own communities of practice.

During an intensive workshop early in the development of narrative medicine at Columbia, we gave a writing prompt to our small group participants: "Write a condolence letter to someone close to you." When it came time for participants in my small group to read aloud to one another what they had written, one of them asked permission to read in a language other than English. Permission was readily granted by the group. The participant read us a letter to his mother in a language that none of us understood and that yet communicated the deepest sense of loss and love and presence and hope. Shmuel's Hebrew expressed what his words could not say. This book that he has co-created with Adina and Wayne continues those early shared efforts to reach, to express, to join with, and to undergo the losses and strengths of others, all of us fellow mortals, all of us committed to healing.

Introduction

....

The hidden patient: An incident that changed my professional life

"Doctor, Nurse Sarah asks that you come quickly. Something bad happened at the Ackermans' home."

That was the entreaty by the man standing at our door at 2 a.m. on a winter's night. Telling him that I would come immediately, I dressed warmly, took my doctor's bag and rushed to my Jeep.

On the way to the nearby farming settlement in rural Israel (about twelve kilometers over a rough, muddy road) I had time to reflect about the Ackermans. Almost two months previously, a middle-aged couple had moved from their cooperative community (kibbutz) to Ni Ya, one of the five agricultural villages in Israel that I served as a physician. The husband had suffered a myocardial infarction and had been hospitalized for three weeks. On discharge, he and his wife had come straight to their new apartment on the Ni Ya grounds, whose clinic I visited every week for two, four-to-five-hour sessions (in addition to being on 24-hour call for emergencies).

The community had a resident nurse (Sarah) who was experienced and efficient. I knew that if she was calling me in the middle of the night it must be an emergency, so I responded without asking the messenger for any details. I had visited Mr. Ackerman in his apartment almost every time I worked at Ni Ya – a total of about ten home visits before that emergency call. Each time, I found no evidence of any organic complications. However, he continued to complain of weakness and light-headedness. Despite the efforts of his wife, the nurse, and myself, he spent most of the day in bed or sitting in a chair. At each visit, his wife was present and asked detailed questions about diet, sleep, bowel habits, etc., often writing down my answers. …

DOI: 10.1201/9781003507529-1

During the drive, I kept visualizing different scenarios. Mr. Ackerman had a recurrent infarct, or perhaps I had missed a cardiac aneurysm that had burst. Had he perhaps developed a deep vein thrombosis in his legs from inactivity and shot a pulmonary embolus? All my scenarios ended in Mr. Ackerman being *in extremis*, if not dead. My own anxiety was high by the time I reached their apartment.

As I entered, the first person I noticed was Mr. Ackerman. To my amazement, he was standing up, came quickly over to me and whispered, "I'm all right, it's my wife!"

Nurse Sarah then quickly took me by the arm and led me into the next room where Mrs. Ackerman was stretched out on the bed. I was dimly aware of Sarah talking to me as I bent over and concentrated on the battered, blood-spattered person on the bed. It took only a few moments to realize that she was dead. Then Sarah's message came into focus – Mrs. Ackerman had committed suicide by throwing herself off a nearby cliff!

Although many years have passed since the incident, I still get a strange feeling when thinking about it. I had been to the Ackermans' home numerous times, always concentrating on the biomedical aspects of the man who had a myocardial infarction, and never paying attention to or noticing the person who was really in need of help!

Following the autopsy and funeral (which the husband attended) there was a mourning period of a week, and then the husband (the same man who until then had reluctantly left his bed) returned to his usual occupation of driving a tractor or plow for a full working day!

All this wreaked havoc on my self-confidence. First, I had missed noticing the really sick person. Second, the original patient, whom I had been unable to get to move from his bed, now, following his wife's death, had returned spontaneously to a full working day! My good biomedical education had not helped me. I had completely missed the dysfunctional family relationship!

The next event in this saga occurred about two weeks later. It was the custom then that every other Friday morning many community physicians would accompany the Chairman of Internal Medicine on a ward round at the nearby university hospital. Following the round, we would adjourn to a small conference room where one or two community physicians would present interesting "cases" for discussion. At the meeting following the suicide incident, I told the story of the "A" couple. There was a short, hushed silence, then the Professor, presumably trying to be kind to me, said, "Dr. Medalie, don't be so upset. After all, the woman was not your patient!"

The Professor's support did not make me feel much better, and the incident occupied my thinking for a long time. After recovering from the shock, I started asking myself what lessons could be learned from this experience. What changes could I introduce to my practice so that this type of situation would not recur?

The unfortunate incident related above was what some call an "Ah-ha" experience. It changed my way of thinking and practicing medicine for all time. After the incident, I became a dedicated proponent of what George Engel called the biopsychosocial model of disease and medical practice.

After much thought, the "hidden patient" concept crystallized: In any family in which there is an individual with an acute, life-threatening or chronic, long-term illness or disease, the caregiver (usually the spouse or the oldest daughter) is under considerable stress. Unless this caregiver receives sufficient support from the family and/or others, coping mechanisms will fail, and the caregiver will develop overt or covert signs of illness—from duodenal ulcers, hypertension and migraine to heart attacks, strokes, and even death.

The incident also impacted me on a personal level. I left the patient's home after filling out the death certificate, etc., at about 4 a.m. I traveled back along a dark country road with the sea on one side and hills on the other. Suddenly I realized that tears were rolling down my cheeks. I stopped the Jeep, turned out the lights and sat in the darkness mouthing, "Mother, Mother."

After a few minutes I asked myself why I was crying. I had been in the Army (Commando Unit) and seen people killed and wounded without crying, and here I was, crying and remembering my mother whom I had last seen some twenty years earlier when, as a seven-year-old boy, I saw her in an open casket at her funeral. She died of cancer of the breast.

The suicide of Mrs. Ackerman had triggered my memory of my mother, and allowed me to grieve, which I had not done until then. … Whatever the reason, this incident changed my life in many ways.[1,2]

* * *

The late **Jack Medalie** narrator of this opening story, qualifies it as a life-changing event, one which transformed him into a practitioner who dared to think outside the box. Carefully challenging dogmas with deep respect for the impact of familial relationships, Medalie further consolidated his biopsychosocial approach. His narrative became an inspirational beacon for the generations of physicians he and his students were molding worldwide. Medalie's story also illuminates a profound transition in his personal trajectory and exemplifies the focus of this book: how physicians are formed and what trajectory their professional life cycle follows. Is it a gradual cumulative growth or one of discrete transitions?

1   Hill, J. (2003). The hidden patient. *Lancet, 362*(9396), 1682. https://doi.org/10.1016/S0140-6736(03)14820-9

2   Medalie, J. H. (1999). The hidden patient: An incident that changed my professional life. In J. M. Borkan, S. Reis, J. H. Medalie, & D. Steinmetz (Eds.), *Patients and doctors: Life-changing stories from primary care.* University of Wisconsin Press. Reproduced with permission.

I AM A DOCTOR, AM I FORTUNATE?

"I AM a doctor" is the proud assertion of a physician who has achieved the desired status after long and arduous years of study.[3] However, what does "I AM a doctor" mean? In the following decades of a medical career, how will this identity evolve? How will it interact with additional identities (family member, citizen)? How stable and unitary (or fluid and multiple) is this identity? What will make the individual a great doctor?[4] What are the milestones and are there prescribed transitions in this trajectory? Does the proud physician ponder, "Who am I, now that I AM a doctor?" And will she return to this pondering over the coming years?

There is a remarkable volume of work on physician training and life. Major advances in the understanding of learning, teaching, and assessment throughout all stages of the professional life cycle have been achieved.[5,6,7,8,9] Bold educational innovations in basic, graduate, and postgraduate medical education have been implemented.[10] The COVID-19 pandemic transformed life and healthcare around the globe and shook multiple assumptions, roles, and behaviors once taken for granted.[11] However, the measured contribution of these understandings, innovations, and disruptions in shaping future physicians is still largely unknown. In other words, despite the wealth of available knowledge, we still lack a well-elaborated description of physician formation and the

3   Frost, H. D., & Regehr, G. (2013). "I am a doctor": Negotiating the discourses of standardization and diversity in professional identity construction. *Academic Medicine: Journal of the Association of American Medical Colleges, 88*(10), 1570–1571. https://doi.org/10.1097/ACM.0b013e3182a34b05

4   Epstein, R. (2017). *Attending: Medicine, mindfulness, and humanity* (1st ed.). Scribner.

5   Knowles, M. S., Holton III, E. F., Swanson, R. A., & Robinson, P. A. (2020). *The adult learner: The definitive classic in adult education and human resource development* (9th ed.). Routledge. https://doi.org/10.4324/9780429299612

6   Knox, A. B. (1977). *Adult development and learning: A handbook on individual growth and competence in the adult years.* Jossey-Bass.

7   Cooke, M., Irby, D. M., & O'Brien, B. C. (2010). *Educating physicians: A call for reform of medical school and residency.* Jossey-Bass.

8   Bleakley, A., Bligh, J., & Browne, J. (2011). *Medical education for the future: Identity, power and location.* Springer.

9   Swanwick, T., Forrest, K., & O'Brien, B. C. (Eds.). (2019). *Understanding medical education: Evidence, theory and practice* (3rd ed.). Wiley-Blackwell.

10 Lucey, C. R., & Johnston, S. C. (2020). The transformational effects of COVID-19 on medical education. *JAMA, 324*(11), 1033–1034. https://doi.org/10.1001/jama.2020.14136

11 Kinnear, B., Zhou, C., Kinnear, B., Carraccio, C., & Schumacher, D. J. (2021). Professional identity formation during the COVID-19 pandemic. *Journal of Hospital Medicine, 16*(1), 44–46. https://doi.org/10.12788/jhm.3540

professional life cycle. Also lacking is a comprehensive theory that may explain it.

The lived experience of this life cycle is conveyed through physician memoirs and other physician-focused narratives, a genre that enjoys exponential growth.[12,13,14] Take, for example, *A Fortunate Man*, first published in 1967.[15,16] Written by **John Berger** and accompanied by endearing black-and-white photography by **Jean Mohr**, the book tells the story of **Dr. John Sassall** (a pseudonym for **Dr. John Eskell**), a British country GP. The following quotes from this masterpiece describe how Sassall's sense of physician identity changed over the years:

> He began to realize that he must face his imagination, even explore it. It must no longer lead always to the "unimaginable" … or, as in his case, to his contemplating only fights within the jaws of death itself. … He began to realize that imagination had to be lived with on every level: his own imagination first – because otherwise this could distort his observation – and then the imagination of his patients.[15]
>
> (pp. 56–57)

> He cures others to cure himself. … Previously the sense of mastery which Sassall gained was the result of the skill with which he dealt with emergencies. … He remained the central character. Now the patient is the central character. … His sense of mastery is fed by the ideal of striving towards the *universal*.[15]
>
> (p. 77)

> Sassall is nevertheless a man doing what he wants. Or, to be more accurate, a man pursuing what he wishes to pursue. Sometimes the pursuit involves strain and disappointment, but in itself it is his unique source of satisfaction. Like an artist or like anybody else who believes that his work justifies his life, Sassall – by our society's miserable standards – is a fortunate man.[15]
>
> (p. 147)

---

12 Moniz, T., Lingard, L., & Watling, C. (2017). Stories doctors tell. *JAMA, 318*(2), 124–125. https://doi.org/10.1001/jama.2017.5518

13 Kalanithi, P. (2016). *When breath becomes air*. Random House.

14 Mostwin, J. (2018). Life-writing from medicine: Biographies and memoirs of physicians. *MedEdPublish (2016), 7*, 196. https://doi.org/10.15694/mep.2018.0000196.1

15 Berger, J., & Mohr, J. (1997). *A fortunate man: The story of a country doctor* (1st ed.). Vintage.

16 Loxterkamp, D. (2013). *What matters in medicine: Lessons from a life in primary care*. The University of Michigan Press.

In his book, Berger summons us to soul search for this quality of "a fortunate man" (or woman). He spells out implicit components of the doctor's journey: imagination (the physician's own and that of his patients), mastery (first for emergencies, second for people), healing oneself while healing others, strain and disappointment, relationships, and dedication. There is more to the story of Sassall—or, rather, Eskell. We revisit it later in this chapter and in Chapter 6.

THE HOUSE OF GOD AND THE ILLNESS NARRATIVES

In striking contrast to *A Fortunate Man* stands **Samuel Shem**'s novel, *The House of God*, celebrating 45 years since it became a must-read for the physician-in-training (us included).[17,18] It is a wild, cynical, gut-wrenching account of the brutal experiences of interns at a top-notch Boston hospital. Later, Shem published *Man's 4th Best Hospital* on the 40th anniversary of *The House of God*, sending the original cast of characters into the recent reality of the US healthcare system, dominated by corporations and digital screens.[19] The result is a similarly brutal account, entirely uncynical, depressing with a glimmer of light at the end of the tunnel (we would hate to spoil the ending).

Back to Berger's focus on the doctor's journey and characteristics, in his seminal *The Illness Narratives*,[20] **Arthur Kleinman** asserts:

> Externalist academic accounts, for all their analytical power, leave something out that is of vital salience for them: namely, the internal, felt experience of doctoring, the story of what it is like to be a healer. ... The ethnography of the physician's care lags far behind the phenomenological description of the experience of illness.
>
> (p. 210)

Whether the protagonist is a British GP in the 1960s, American interns in the 1980s, or their mature selves in the 2010s, Kleinman's words mirror a sentiment present in the aforementioned books and still hold true today. With this view in mind, Kleinman quotes a practitioner who "tells us that becoming a healer resolved a key tension in his adolescent

---

17 Shem, S. (2010). *The house of God*. Berkley.
18 Kohn, M., & Donley, C. (Eds.). (2008). *Return to the house of God: Medical resident education 1978–2008*. The Kent State University Press.
19 Shem, S. (2019). *Man's 4th best hospital*. Berkley.
20 Kleinman, A. (1989). *The illness narratives: Suffering, healing, and the human condition*. Basic Books.

development and adult personality," echoing Berger. Regarding this quoted physician and another interviewed doctor, Kleinman writes: "Both practitioners see themselves as students of human nature, teachers of moral wisdom."

BACK TO THE FUTURE, *A FORTUNATE WOMAN*

In the foreword to *Medical Education for the Future* by **Bleakley** et al., **Hodges** claims that "the staunchly individualist hero-doctor is no longer the ideal. Medical education instead aims to develop medical professionals who can participate in dispersed social networks that form and reform to accomplish clearly defined healthcare goals." Bleakley et al., Hodges, and others point to learning during the doctor's life cycle as a social act embedded within a community of practice rather than a solitary trajectory.

In mid-2022, *A Fortunate Woman* by **Polly Morland** was published, revisiting Berger's account from 1967.[21] In its pages, Morland relates her story as a female GP in the same practice that Dr. John Eskell established. The book is a striking illustration of the changes that have taken place over half a century in rural United Kingdom general practice, but also of considerable universal similarities. First, as two-thirds of United Kingdom GPs are now women, so too the protagonist is fittingly female. Second, consultations are now by appointment, and 24/7 availability is now shared and sometimes delegated. Third, computers have replaced hand-written records and cellular phones have replaced the old dial telephones, introducing remote consultations that became so handy during the COVID-19 pandemic (the impact of which is also described in Morland's book). Fourth, Morland is well-rooted professionally in a community of practice: she has been practicing medicine for over 20 years, having begun with Eskell's original practice partner; she has in-practice trainees, a well-established support team with multiple skills, and firm contacts with the regional and national professional network, which includes her writing for a GP journal. Fifth, she carries the torch that Eskell exemplified: the utmost importance of patient–physician relationships, deep knowledge of patients and their context and stories, a few house calls each day, and the particular clinical method that is appropriate for this discipline.

Most scholarly and literary attention has been directed at the medical school years,[22] much to the following residency (vocational training)

---

21 Morland, P. (2022). *A fortunate woman: A country doctor's story*. Picador.

22 Poirier, S. (2006). Medical education and the embodied physician. *Literature and Medicine*, 25(2), 522–552. https://doi.org/10.1353/lm.2007.0008

period,[23] and there is now also some growing interest in the longest season of the physician's life—the years in practice.[24] Tentatively, an integrative gaze that contains all three of these phases, rare until a decade ago, is emerging. Discourses around competence and professionalism,[25] competency-based education,[26] lifelong learning,[27] expertise,[28] and reflection and narrative have recently become integrated under the construct of professional identity formation.[29] As this transition becomes more visible, we see this time as an opportune moment to take stock of this issue, drawing out a more concrete, organized, and encompassing view of the physician's life cycle.

While reflecting on our own development and that of our teachers, students, and colleagues, as well as immersing ourselves in the literature, we read about and identified in ourselves a series of transitions that guide an emergent practitioner's trajectory.[30,31] What are the characteristics of these transitional experiences? Can they be taught and embedded into an educational context? Are there passages common to all learners in medicine? Is the clearer understanding of professional identity formation

23 Wright, S. M., Levine, R. B., Beasley, B., Haidet, P., Gress, T. W., Caccamese, S., Brady, D., Marwaha, A., & Kern, D. E. (2006). Personal growth and its correlates during residency training. *Medical Education, 40*(8), 737–745. https://doi.org/10.1111/j.1365-2929.2006.02499.x

24 Davis, D. A., Barnes, B., & Fox, R. D. (2003). *The continuing professional development of physicians: From research to practice.* AMA Press.

25 Cruess, R. L., Cruess, S. R., & Steinert, Y. (Eds.). (2016). *Teaching medical professionalism: Supporting the development of a professional identity* (2nd ed.). Cambridge University Press.

26 Epstein, R. M., & Hundert, E. M. (2002). Defining and assessing professional competence. *JAMA, 287*(2), 226–235. https://doi.org/10.1001/jama.287.2.226

27 Albanese, M. A. (2006). Crafting the reflective lifelong learner: Why, what and how. *Medical Education, 40*(4), 288–290. https://doi.org/10.1111/j.1365-2929.2006.02470.x

28 Dunphy, B. C., & Williamson, S. L. (2004). In pursuit of expertise: Toward an educational model for expertise development. *Advances in Health Sciences Education: Theory and Practice, 9*(2), 107–127. https://doi.org/10.1023/B:AHSE.0000027436.17220.9c

29 Wald, H. S. (2015). Professional identity (trans) formation in medical education: Reflection, relationship, resilience. *Academic Medicine: Journal of the Association of American Medical Colleges, 90*(6), 701–706. https://doi.org/10.1097/ACM.0000000000000731

30 Volpe, R. L., Hopkins, M., Haidet, P., Wolpaw, D. R., & Adams, N. E. (2019). Is research on professional identity formation biased? Early insights from a scoping review and metasynthesis. *Medical Education, 53*(2), 119–132. https://doi.org/10.1111/medu.13781

31 Sugarman, L. (1986). *Life-span development: Concepts, theories and interventions.* Routledge.

in the last two decades supporting a more coherent development? These were some of the questions that puzzled us as we embarked on the journey of writing this book. Once more, we quote Kleinman: "What is important is to lay out the anatomy of successful healing so that it can be understood, taught, acquired, and more routinely practiced" (p. 226).

Berger, Morland, and Kleinman all describe advanced professionals who embody "successful healing." The "average physician" may not live up to these standards. Most of the literature retrieved echoes this, addressing aspirations for the fully mature professional, who is almost ideal, always heroic, and larger than life. Examples of "partial healers" and some "failed healers" prevail.[32] In addition, bias, discrimination (such as gender- or race-based), and abuse are ubiquitous in medicine. The dominance of white, male physicians (at least in North America) is both being challenged and radically changing. The life cycle of women and Black physicians in medicine is fundamentally influenced by their identities and warrants special attention. As **Volpe** et al.[33] assert, the entire medical education literature on the doctor's life cycle and professional identity formation may well be biased by largely ignoring these issues.

Finally, the physician's role, job description, and reality have changed dramatically in recent decades, a process further compounded by the coronavirus pandemic. This is especially apparent when compared with the medical world of Eskell 55–75 years ago. While the enduring values of the medical profession[34] seem to prevail, the digital age, precision medicine and "omics" technologies, globalization, bureaucratization of medicine,[35] the awakening to the role of gender, race, and ethnicity as well as bias, discrimination, and mistreatment, and finally the COVID-19 pandemic, to name a few, challenge the sustainability of humanism and professionalism, reveal hitherto hidden aspects, and render lifelong learning increasingly challenging. The doctor's life cycle is transforming even as we write these lines.

---

32 Candilis, P. J., & Sulmasy, L. S. (2019). Physician impairment and rehabilitation. *Annals of Internal Medicine*, 171(9), 681–682. https://doi.org/10.7326/L19-0554

33 Volpe, R. L., Hopkins, M., Haidet, P., Wolpaw, D. R., & Adams, N. E. (2019). Is research on professional identity formation biased? Early insights from a scoping review and metasynthesis. *Medical Education*, 53(2), 119–132. https://doi.org/10.1111/medu.13781

34 Loscalzo, J. L., Fauci, A. S., Kasper, D. L., Hauser, S. L., Longo, D. L., & Jameson, J. L. (Eds.). (2022). *Harrison's principles of internal medicine* (21st ed.). McGraw-Hill.

35 Ludmerer, K. M. (2015). *Let me heal: The opportunity to preserve excellence in American medicine*. Oxford University Press.

LITERATURE SEARCH AND FINDINGS

We searched the literature (up to the end of February 2024; see the Appendix for our search strategy), consulted experts, and summarized our own experiences in the domain of becoming and being a physician. Then, we embarked on an iterative consensus process, more intuitive than formal, of categorizing our findings. Over several years, this process first yielded categories 1–5 and 9, and subsequently categories 6–8, resulting in nine categories encompassing the doctor's life cycle:

1. Developmental theories: stages, transitions, and liminality
2. Adult learning and continuous medical education: the practice years
3. Expertise, clinical reasoning, deliberate practice, and phronesis
4. Moral and character development
5. Narrative, storytelling, and reflection: the handling of emotions
6. Developmental issues, remediation, and the wounded healer
7. Gender, race, and core identities: bias, discrimination, and mistreatment in medicine
8. The impact of COVID-19 on the doctor's life cycle
9. Professional identity formation: incorporating professionalism and care

In other words, our inquiry had a complex life cycle of its own, with emergent insights unfolding along the way.

This book is both a description of each category and an attempt to synthesize them. Each chapter is dedicated to a category and, as in this introduction, opens with a relevant narrative to humanize the scholarly text and at times introduce additional dimensions. In the Discussion (Chapter 10), we present an outline of the emergent state-of-the-art synergistic view of the doctor's life cycle discourse and conclude with suggestions for future directions aimed at informing a relevant education and research agenda in the years to come.

REFERENCES

Albanese, M. A. (2006). Crafting the reflective lifelong learner: Why, what and how. *Medical Education*, 40(4), 288–290. https://doi.org/10.1111/j.1365-2929.2006.02470.x

Berger, J., & Mohr, J. (1997). *A fortunate man: The story of a country doctor* (1st ed.). Vintage.

Bleakley, A., Bligh, J., & Browne, J. (2011). *Medical education for the future: Identity, power and location.* Springer.

Candilis, P. J., & Sulmasy, L. S. (2019). Physician impairment and rehabilitation. *Annals of Internal Medicine*, 171(9), 681–682. https://doi.org/10.7326/L19-0554

Cooke, M., Irby, D. M., & O'Brien, B. C. (2010). *Educating physicians: A call for reform of medical school and residency.* Jossey-Bass.

Cruess, R. L., Cruess, S. R., & Steinert, Y. (Eds.). (2016). *Teaching medical professionalism: Supporting the development of a professional identity* (2nd ed.). Cambridge University Press.

Davis, D. A., Barnes, B., & Fox, R. D. (2003). *The continuing professional development of physicians: From research to practice*. AMA Press.

Dunphy, B. C., & Williamson, S. L. (2004). In pursuit of expertise: Toward an educational model for expertise development. *Advances in Health Sciences Education: Theory and Practice*, 9(2), 107–127. https://doi.org/10.1023/B:AHSE .0000027436.17220.9c

Epstein, R. M. (2017). *Attending: Medicine, mindfulness, and humanity* (1st ed.). Scribner.

Epstein, R. M., & Hundert, E. M. (2002). Defining and assessing professional competence. *JAMA*, 287(2), 226–235. https://doi.org/10.1001/jama.287.2.226

Frost, H. D., & Regehr, G. (2013). "I am a doctor": Negotiating the discourses of standardization and diversity in professional identity construction. *Academic Medicine: Journal of the Association of American Medical Colleges*, 88(10), 1570–1571. https://doi.org/10.1097/ACM.0b013e3182a34b05

Hill, J. (2003). The hidden patient. *Lancet*, 362(9396), 1682. https://doi.org/10.1016/ S0140-6736(03)14820-9

Kalanithi, P. (2016). *When breath becomes air*. Random House.

Kinnear, B., Zhou, C., Kinnear, B., Carraccio, C., & Schumacher, D. J. (2021). Professional identity formation during the COVID-19 pandemic. *Journal of Hospital Medicine*, 16(1), 44–46. https://doi.org/10.12788/jhm.3540

Kleinman, A. (1989). *The illness narratives: Suffering, healing, and the human condition*. Basic Books.

Knowles, M. S., Holton III, E. F., Swanson, R. A., & Robinson, P. A. (2020). *The adult learner: The definitive classic in adult education and human resource development* (9th ed.). Routledge. https://doi.org/10.4324/9780429299612

Knox, A. B. (1977). *Adult development and learning: A handbook on individual growth and competence in the adult years*. Jossey-Bass.

Kohn, M., & Donley, C. (Eds.). (2008). *Return to the house of God: Medical resident education 1978–2008*. The Kent State University Press.

Loscalzo, J. L., Fauci, A. S., Kasper, D. L., Hauser, S. L., Longo, D. L., & Jameson, J. L. (Eds.). (2022). *Harrison's principles of internal medicine* (21st ed.). McGraw-Hill.

Loxterkamp, D. (2013). *What matters in medicine: Lessons from a life in primary care*. The University of Michigan Press.

Lucey, C. R., & Johnston, S. C. (2020). The transformational effects of COVID-19 on medical education. *JAMA*, 324(11), 1033–1034. https://doi.org/10.1001/jama.2020 .14136

Ludmerer, K. M. (2015). *Let me heal: The opportunity to preserve excellence in American medicine*. Oxford University Press.

Medalie, J. H. (1999). The hidden patient: An incident that changed my professional life. In J. M. Borkan, S. Reis, J. H. Medalie, & D. Steinmetz (Eds.), *Patients and doctors: Life-changing stories from primary care*. University of Wisconsin Press.

Moniz, T., Lingard, L., & Watling, C. (2017). Stories doctors tell. *JAMA*, 318(2), 124–125. https://doi.org/10.1001/jama.2017.5518

Morland, P. (2022). *A fortunate woman: A country doctor's story*. Picador.

Mostwin, J. (2018). Life-writing from medicine: Biographies and memoirs of physicians. *MedEdPublish (2016)*, 7, 196. https://doi.org/10.15694/mep.2018.0000196.1

Poirier, S. (2006). Medical education and the embodied physician. *Literature and Medicine*, 25(2), 522–552. https://doi.org/10.1353/lm.2007.0008

Shem, S. (2010). *The house of God*. Berkley.

Shem, S. (2019). *Man's 4th best hospital*. Berkley.

Stewart, M., Brown, J. B., Weston, W. W., Freeman, T., Ryan, B. L., McWilliam, C. L., & McWhinney, I. R. (2024). *Patient-centered medicine: Transforming the clinical method* (4th ed.). CRC Press.

Sugarman, L. (1986). *Life-span development: Concepts, theories and interventions.* Routledge.

Swanwick, T., Forrest, K., & O'Brien, B. C. (Eds.). (2019). *Understanding medical education: Evidence, theory and practice* (3rd ed.). Wiley-Blackwell.

Volpe, R. L., Hopkins, M., Haidet, P., Wolpaw, D. R., & Adams, N. E. (2019). Is research on professional identity formation biased? Early insights from a scoping review and metasynthesis. *Medical Education, 53*(2), 119–132. https://doi.org/10.1111/medu.13781

Wald, H. S. (2015). Professional identity (trans) formation in medical education: Reflection, relationship, resilience. *Academic Medicine: Journal of the Association of American Medical Colleges, 90*(6), 701–706. https://doi.org/10.1097/ACM.0000000000000731

Wright, S. M., Levine, R. B., Beasley, B., Haidet, P., Gress, T. W., Caccamese, S., Brady, D., Marwaha, A., & Kern, D. E. (2006). Personal growth and its correlates during residency training. *Medical Education, 40*(8), 737–745. https://doi.org/10.1111/j.1365-2929.2006.02499.x

CHAPTER 1

Developmental theories

Stages, transitions, and liminality

....

Wild Strawberries

The movie *Wild Strawberries* is a masterpiece by Ingmar Bergman. … The film is ostensibly about an elderly physician, Isak Borg, who is to receive an academic award for his life of achievement within medical practice. A widower, he is somewhat estranged from his only son and his daughter-in-law, who announces during the film that she is pregnant. The story is of his journey to receive the award, of his looking back on his life as he progresses towards the public recognition of the event, of the people he meets on the way … and of the dreams that he has, and the growth and development that ensues.

Most interesting is the dream Borg has in which he is alone on a street and comes upon a hearse and a casket which falls open, revealing the corpse to be himself while a clock on a side pole melts. He is horrified in the dream and upon awakening. The dream seems to indicate a partial recognition that he himself is a dead man walking. He is dead inside; his capacity for love is dead. He is frozen in time even as time passes because he has not grown as a person. The film then becomes a journey of self-revealing memory. … He is portrayed then as a rigid young man, self-centered, with a stern moralism used as justification for his sense of superiority.

What is the ability to love, asks the film. How does it develop? What is its relationship to human relationships and to moral values? Is there still time for this elderly man to learn to love? Was he able to love in his work as a physician? …

DOI: 10.1201/9781003507529-2

In the next dream, Borg is both his present elderly self yet also a student being quizzed by another physician, who is excoriatingly abusive. In the dream, he does not know the answer to the inquisitor's first two factual questions. The third question is what a physician's first duty is. He answers with the classic to do no harm. He is contemptuously told that there is a higher duty: to beg forgiveness. ...

Most interesting and touching is the elderly housekeeper who has been devoted to him as a mother or as a good doctor is to a patient. It is a devotion of consistency and reliability, as a form of duty but also as a form of love for the real patient and the real craft of caregiving. ... The end of the story shows him the night after his award, being tucked in by the old woman housekeeper. He finally wishes to thank her and to express his love for her. ... The film thus ends with perhaps the possibility of a more relaxed and real human relationship.[1]

* * *

ORIGINS OF PHYSICIAN LIFESPAN GROWTH AND DEVELOPMENT THEORIES

Lifespan growth and development have preoccupied multiple scholars.[2,3,4,5] The concept derives from biology: an orderly progression in which more complex forms are created by the differentiation and reintegration of earlier simpler forms.[6] Its study was most salient during the third quarter of the last century and is associated with a psychodynamic approach. Scholars of lifespan development are often popularized and enjoy wide publicity (**Sheehy, Levinson**). Probably the best known of these scholars is **Erik Erikson**, who described a sequenced, staged model of human development from birth to death through eight periods; each requires a distinct developmental task, polarized into dysfunctional and functional stances. Erikson published a paper in which he analyzed *Wild Strawberries*, a fine example of his model applied to the physician life cycle. In the present chapter, the opening account about the movie is by **Eric Marcus,** a psychiatrist who describes the film from a more psychoanalytic stance.

1   Marcus, E. R. (2013). Wild strawberries. *Bulletin of the Association for Psychoanalytic Medicine*, 2(1), 45–58. Reproduced with permission of the author.
2   Erikson, E. H. (1968). *Identity, youth and crisis*. W.W. Norton Company.
3   Sheehy, G. (2006). *Passages: Predictable crises in adult life* (30th Anniversary ed.). Ballantine Books.
4   Levinson, D. J. (1980). Toward a conception of the adult life course. In N. J. Smelser (Ed.), *Themes of work and love in adulthood*. Harvard University Press.
5   Erikson, E. H. (1976). Reflections on Dr. Borg's life cycle. *Daedalus*, *105*(2), 1–28.
6   Sugarman, L. (1986). *Life-span development: Concepts, theories and interventions*. Routledge.

Universal issues emerge: a physician's life cycle, love and duty, relationships and moral values, and the interplay of the personal and professional.

One of the earliest publications addressing the development of a professional identity among medical students is *The Student-Physician*, published in 1957 and edited by **Merton** et al.[7] Merton writes:

> It is their function [of medical schools] to transmit the culture of medicine and to advance that culture. It is their task to shape the novice into the effective practitioner of medicine, to give him the best available knowledge and skills, and to provide him with a professional identity so that he comes to think, act, and feel like a physician.
>
> (p. 7)

This vision has come full circle since the 1950s and is currently being revisited and expanded upon.

In one of the book's chapters, "The Development of a Professional Self-Image," **Mary Jean Huntington** reviews the results of a survey of medical students across all four years at three medical schools in the United States. The students were asked: "In the most recent dealings you have had with patients, how have you tended to think of yourself, primarily as a doctor rather than as a student, or primarily as a student rather than as a doctor?" Students increasingly thought of themselves as physicians from the end of their first year (31%) to the end of their fourth year (83%). First-year students were more likely to think of themselves as physicians in dealing with patients (31%), compared to dealing with nurses (12%), classmates (3%), and faculty (2%). These results may have been influenced by the fact that this part of the study was conducted with two classes from Case Western Reserve University School of Medicine, where students were involved in closely following a family from early on in their first year of study. Students whose families presented medical problems showed a greater tendency to develop the self-image of a physician, especially when they felt that they had handled these problems without difficulty.

The first to explicitly associate lifespan development with the formation of physicians was Levinson in a 1967 paper[8] reviewing the book *Boys in White: Student Culture in Medical School*,[9] an ethnographic

7   Merton, R. K., Reader, G. G., & Kendall, P. L. (Eds.). (1957). *The student physician: Introductory studies in the sociology of medical education*. Harvard University Press. http://dx.doi.org/10.4159/harvard.9780674366831

8   Levinson, D. J. (1967). Medical education and the theory of adult socialization. *Journal of Health and Social Behavior, 8*(4), 253–265. https://psycnet.apa.org/doi/10.2307/2948419

9   Becker, H., Geer, B., Hughes, E. C., & Strauss A. L. (1976). *Boys in white: Student culture in medical school* (Reprint ed.). Transaction Publishers.

study of medical students' experiences at a Kansas medical school in the mid- to late-1950s, published six years prior by **Becker** et al. (At the time, nearly all medical school students were male and White. In 2018, the number of female medical students surpassed that of males for the first time in the United States.[10]) Levinson compares the study of Becker et al. with **Renée Fox**'s chapter in *The Student-Physician*, titled "Training for Uncertainty." Fox found evidence that students were moved and often troubled by their experiences in the anatomy lab or at autopsies, stimulating ego defenses in their efforts to find a **balance between detachment and concern** in their relationships with patients. Becker et al., on the other hand, argued that these feelings were quickly brushed aside as students focused on technical competence and grades. For Levinson, the methodology used in the study by Becker et al. excluded any exploration of students' personal feelings or struggles and therefore could not obtain data on psychodynamic aspects of socialization into medicine. *Boys in White* and Levinson's review both mention the first cadaver dissection and first patient death as seminal events for all medical students, introducing **rites of passage** into medical education discourse.

THE DOCTOR TREE

Following the line of psychodynamic-oriented inquiry, a slim volume titled *The Doctor Tree: Developmental Stages in the Growth of Physicians*, published by the psychiatrist/psychologist couple **Ralph Zabarenko** and **Lucy Zabarenko** in 1978, is the earliest we could find to attempt a full description of developmental stages in the growth of physicians.[11] The Zabarenkos' theory is based on extensive observations in medical education as well as their psychodynamic orientation.[12] Opening with a medical error vignette, they subsequently state:

> It seemed plain that doctors develop as they are educated and that such development must have order. We thought of this development as a tangled web of developmental lines among which we could distinguish five that seemed to have sufficient explanatory power.

10 Roberts, L. W. (2020). Women and academic medicine, 2020. *Academic Medicine: Journal of the Association of American Medical Colleges, 95*(10), 1459–1464. https://doi.org/10.1097/ACM.0000000000003617

11 Zabarenko, R. N., & Zabarenko, L. M. (1978). *The doctor tree: Developmental stages in the growth of physicians*. University of Pittsburgh Press.

12 Zabarenko, R. N., Zabarenko, L., & Pittenger, R. A. (1970). The psychodynamics of physicianhood. *Psychiatry, 33*(1), 102–118. https://doi.org/10.1080/00332747.1970.11023617

The Doctor Tree progresses from describing the tree's "roots," which are physicians' core developmental processes, to five developmental stages that are the tree's "branches." Among these roots are "residues of oedipal conflict" (affecting the nurturance–authority poles of medical care); past traumas; a physician's ego-ideal; an objectivity–empathy continuum; and an activation of healing behavior. The five developmental stages are divided into the first three, which belong to earlier development, and the latter two, which are "slower to begin, slower to mature, more rarely approaching the highest levels." These five stages are:

1. Balancing the oscillation between objectivity and empathy (or in present-day terms, **detached concern versus empathy**)
2. Appropriate management of nurturing tendencies and executive necessities (**emotional needs versus performance**)
3. Adequate regulation and control of the need for omnipotence by appropriate appreciation of the realities of medical work, especially those related to tolerance for uncertainty (**tolerance for uncertainty and taming of hubris**)
4. Formation of an internal ideal of physicianhood; that is, a professional ego-ideal (**early professional identity formation [PIF]**)
5. Maturation of an operational professional identity (**mature PIF**)

In *The Doctor Tree*, the Zabarenkos contend that sufficient mastery of para-cognitive factors must coincide with or precede cognitive mastery and be adequate enough to support the latter. This statement is well aligned with present-day recognition of metacognition (thinking about thinking),[13] core competencies in medicine,[14] and the necessity of integrating cognitive growth with attention to emotions. Further, they state their basic assumptions: later development is superimposed upon preceding stages; early growth influences and partly determines subsequent development; and a notion of critical integration and synthesis is achieved when some skills become automatic (as in music or sports), evoking the construct of expertise (see Chapter 3).

The Zabarenkos have not been quoted extensively in the literature. However, the discourse that they initiated is often repeated by later scholars, with many similar metaphors, concerns, constructs, and conclusions.

---

13 Quirk, M. (2006). *Intuition and metacognition in medical education: Keys to developing expertise*. Springer.
14 General Medical Council. (2018). *Outcomes for graduates*. https://www.gmc-uk .org/-/media/documents/dc11326-outcomes-for-graduates-2018_pdf-75040796.pdf

Surprisingly, their fourth and fifth "branches" are very similar to the new buzz phrase in medical education: professional identity formation.

Soon after the release of *The Doctor Tree*, **Brent**,[15] then a psychiatry resident, described residency as a developmental process, quoting the Zabarenkos, Erikson, and Levinson. He adds to the constructs in the physician developmental discourse by identifying conflicts between **vulnerability and invulnerability, active versus passive, and helplessness versus problem solving** as the core resident struggles. **Boundary maintenance and professional identity** are identified as the core tasks. Brent concludes that residency is more than the acquisition of knowledge and skills—it is also about attitudes and self-representations—and summons attention to the developmental processes that will certainly take place through **mentoring, advising, and support groups,** when available.

Almost two decades later, another psychiatrist, Marcus (the author of this chapter's opening piece), reported a study of medical school students' dreams.'[16,17] The report produces stages and characteristics of the developing identity by year of study, from first-year "empathic identity and student-centered humanism" to fourth-year "patient-centered craft identity and craft humanism." In the dreams, Marcus identifies masochistic fantasies, narcissistic rage, and sadistic fantasies, which appear at different stages, indicating the inner struggles students experience throughout their studies.

BEYOND PSYCHODYNAMICS

The next scholars addressing the physician developmental paradigm are from the Department of Family Medicine at Western University (then the University of Western Ontario).[18,19] Based on many years of patient care

---

15 Brent, D. A. (1981). The residency as a developmental process. *Journal of Medical Education*, 56(5), 417–422. https://doi.org/10.1097/00001888-198105000-00006

16 Marcus, E. R. (2003). Medical student dreams about medical school: The unconscious developmental process of becoming a physician. *International Journal of Psycho-Analysis*, 84(Pt 2), 367–386. https://doi.org/10.1516/002075703321632964

17 Marcus, E. R. (1999). Empathy, humanism, and the professionalization process of medical education. *Academic Medicine: Journal of the Association of American Medical Colleges*, 74(11), 1211–1215. https://doi.org/10.1097/00001888-199911000-00014

18 Carroll, J. G., Lipkin, M., Nachtigall, L., & Weston, W. W. (1995). A developmental awareness for teaching doctor/patient communication skills. In M. Lipkin, S. M. Putnam, A. Lazare, J. G. Carroll, & R. M. Frankel (Eds.), *The medical interview* (pp. 388–396). Frontiers of Primary Care. Springer. https://doi.org/10.1007/978-1-4612-2488-4_32

19 Weston, W. W., & Lipkin, M. Jr. (1989). Doctors learning communication skills: Developmental issues. In M. Stewart & D. Roter (Eds.), *Communicating with medical patients* (pp. 43–57). Sage Publications.

and interprofessional collaboration in theory and practice, they offer (in the chapter of a book, now in its fourth edition) a composite description of the stages of physician formation. First, **gaining technical competence:** the principal focus of medical school is the recognition and treatment of disease, which may result in a lack of attention to the human side of medicine. Next is **developing a professional identity**, from clerkships through to residency. Finally, **learning to heal** occurs in the five to ten years following residency and **is not accomplished by all physicians.** This latter stage requires **frequent encouragement, support, effective role modeling, and opportunities to discuss feelings and internal struggles** for the physician to adopt the healer's mantle.

Weston (a co-author of this book) and **Brown** identify four types of helpful scholarly approaches in their quest to understand the professional journey. First is the many personal narratives published in recent decades, in which learners recount their experiences through their formative years. In these texts, the authors make sense of their often-traumatic stories (see, for example, the opening narratives of the Introduction and Chapter 5), which may have desensitized them to human suffering and contributed to their impatience and detachment (dehumanization). Second, Weston and colleagues introduce a developmental theory where a loss of simplicity, especially in the moral development of college students, is described (see Chapter 4). Third is the role of mentoring, where role models offer support, challenge, and provide vision. Fourth, professionalism and professional formation (see Chapter 9) are informed by the exponential interest in this construct in recent decades.[20]

Furthermore, Weston and colleagues describe concrete critical passages such as encountering a cadaver; meeting the first patient; the first intimate physical examination; the first death; graduation; internship, constituting initiation into personal responsibility; specialization; going out into practice; and the long haul of the practice years.

---

20 Weston, W. W., & Brown, J. B. (2024). Becoming a physician: The human experience of medical education. In M. Stewart, J. B. Brown, W. W. Weston, T. R. Freeman, B. L. Ryan, C. L. McWilliam, & I. R. McWhinney (Eds.), *Patient-centered medicine: Transforming the clinical method* (4th ed.). CRC Press.

ROBERT KEGAN'S THEORY OF DEVELOPMENT

Kegan's constructivist developmental theory emerged in the 1980s and has been evolving since.[21] It has been employed in health profession education including dentistry, in the United States military, and in business leadership interventions.[22,23] Kegan posits five stages of consciousness development that progress from the childhood impulsive mind to the instrumental mind, socialized mind, self-authoring mind, and finally the self-transforming mind (Figure 1.1).

Individuals at the **second, instrumental mind** stage:

> Organize events into concrete categories and are able to take the perspective of others. This structure enables them to … construct a stable sense of self and participate in close relationships based on social exchange. … Although individuals at Stage 2 can take the point of view of others and understand their perspectives, they do so in terms of their OWN needs and interests. That is, their own needs become the lens through which they understand their social world.[24]

Regarding those with **socialized minds**:

> The Stage 3 individual is able to organize experiences and events into abstract categories and to view multiple perspectives simultaneously. This new ability allows them to become identified with others; hence,

21 Lewin, L. O., McManamon, A., Stein, M. T. O., & Chen, D. T. (2019). Minding the form that transforms: Using Kegan's model of adult development to understand personal and professional identity formation in medicine. *Academic Medicine: Journal of the Association of American Medical Colleges*, 94(9), 1299–1304. https://doi.org /10.1097/ACM.0000000000002741

22 Kegan, R. (2009). What "form" transforms? A constructive-developmental approach to transformative learning. In K. Illeris (Ed.), *Contemporary theories of learning: Learning theorists in their own words* (pp. 35–54). Routledge.

23 Forsythe, G. B., Snook, S., Lewis, P., & Bartone, P. T. (2002). Making sense of officership: Developing a professional identity for 21st century army officers. In D. M. Snider & G. L. Watkins (Eds.), *The future of the army profession* (pp. 357–378). McGraw-Hill.

24 Forsythe, G. B. (2005). Identity development in professional education. *Academic Medicine: Journal of the Association of American Medical Colleges*, 80(Suppl 10), S112–S117. https://doi.org/10.1097/00001888-200510001-00029

Kegan's Stages of Development	Typical Ages	Associated Traits	Systems in Scope	Object (under conscious control)	Subject (under development)
Impulsive Mind (1st Order Consciousness)	~2–6 years	• idea of "durable objects" un(der)developed • mystified when others have different opinions • need to be repeatedly reminded of rules			one's impulses and perceptions
Instrumental Mind (2nd Order Consciousness)	~6 yrs–teens; (& some adults)	• tendency to view relationships in utilitarian terms • limited ability to take other's perspectives • seeks out and follows unchanging, universal rules		one's impulses and perceptions	one's needs, interests, desires
Socialized Mind (3rd Order Consciousness)	post-teens (& most adults)	• oriented to maintaining affiliation with one's "tribe" • capable of goal setting, planning, self-reflection • able to think abstractly and reflect on others' actions		one's needs, interests, desires	interpersonal relationships, mutuality
Self-Authoring Mind (4th Order Consciousness)	variable (~35% of adults)	• identifies values and aims to contribute meaningfully • able to recognize need for and to nurture affiliations • self-guided, self-evaluative, and responsible		interpersonal relationships, mutuality	self-authorship, identity, ideology
Self-Transforming Mind (5th Order Consciousness)	variable (<1% of adults)	• able to regard multiple ideologies simultaneously • able to think systemically and embrace complexity • attentive to multiple levels (self, collective, systemic)		self-authorship, identity, ideology	dialectic among ideologies

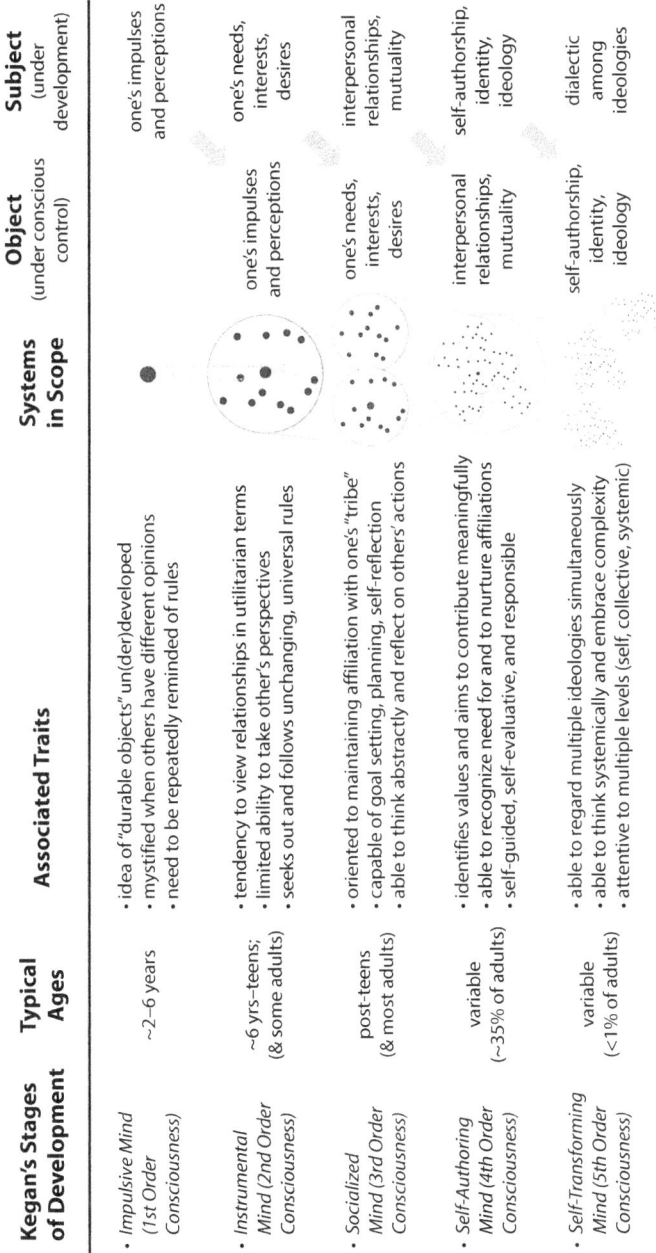

FIGURE 1.1 Kegan's Stages of Development (Reproduced with permission. Davis, B., & Francis, K. 2024. "Constructive-Developmental Theory" in *Discourses on Learning in Education*. https://learningdiscourses.com.)

interpersonal mutuality emerges. ... Put another way, at Stage 3, we become our relationships; we experience a shared identity at Stage 3 rather than a personal identity. With regard to professional identity, it's as if Stage 3 individuals "are the profession"; they are fully bought in and take on all the expectations of the profession. The limitation, however, is that they are unable to reconcile competing expectations because they have not yet "integrated" the expectations of the profession into their own sense of self.

At the **self-authoring stage:**

We can take a perspective on relationships and assess them in terms of self-authored principles and standards. The transition from Stage 3 to Stage 4 is the story of moving from "being relationships" to "having relationships." Stage 4 is about psychological autonomy. Self-generated values and principles provide a perspective on one's relationships; the shift is from shared expectations to personal expectations. ... From a professional perspective, Stage 4 individuals have internalized and personalized the values and expectations of the profession—they are able [to] articulate the relationship among expectations, and they "own" them as their own. Violations of such expectations bring a sense of violations of one's internal standards, not simply the violation of what others expect.

The **self-transforming stage:**

Is never seen before midlife and is seen only rarely then. ... Adults at the Fifth Order are less likely to see the world in terms of dichotomies or polarities. They are more likely to understand and deal well with paradox and with managing the tension of opposites. ... They are more likely to consider the advantages not just of other opinions ... but of entirely different forms of governing systems. They may realize that their internal system itself contributes to their inability to perceive a wide enough field of alternatives.[25]

In other words, they embrace transformations.

Kegan's framework has been used extensively with the understanding that "when we encounter professional error and mistake, it often has less to do with knowledge and skills than it has to do with

---

25 Berger, J. G. (2002). A summary of the constructive-developmental theory of Robert Kegan.

the maturity, judgement, values, and professionalism. These outcomes matter."[26] **Rule** and **Bebeau**, for example, adopted Kegan's framework in a book that celebrates dentists' inspiring stories of professional commitment.[27] Recently, the model was applied in basic medical education (BME) by co-author of this book **Adina Kalet** and coworkers, who assessed each subject's stage of development in various studies through analysis of interviews and narratives written in response to structured questions.[28]

In the current wave of developmental discourse, **Jarvis-Selinger** et al.[29] were among the first to write about PIF. They distinguish between **individual and collective identities** using Kegan's stage model to describe individual identity formation. Further, they emphasize that **transitions in this journey are not gradual**, but rather "marked by abrupt discontinuities" and "precipitated by emerging 'crises.'"[30] Transitions serve as turning points where the individual also experiences increased vulnerability.

WHAT PHYSICIANS FIND MEANINGFUL AND HEALING IN THEIR WORK

The latest wave of discourse on the physician life cycle has introduced additional perspectives, including the role of emotions, physician wellbeing,[31] and what physicians find meaningful and healing in their

26 Forsythe, G. B. (2005). Identity development in professional education. *Academic Medicine: Journal of the Association of American Medical Colleges, 80*(Suppl 10), S112–S117. https://doi.org/10.1097/00001888-200510001-00029

27 Rule, J. T., & Bebeau, M. J. (2005). *Dentists who care: Inspiring stories of professional commitment.* Quintessence Books.

28 Kalet, A., Ark, T. K., Monson, V., Song, H. S., Buckvar-Keltz, L., Harnik, V., Yingling, S., Rivera, R., Jr, Tewksbury, L., Lusk, P., & Crowe, R. (2021). Does a measure of medical professional identity formation predict communication skills performance? *Patient Education and Counseling, 104*(12), 3045–3052. https://doi.org/10.1016/j.pec.2021.03.040

29 Jarvis-Selinger, S., Pratt, D. D., & Regehr, G. (2012). Competency is not enough: Integrating identity formation into the medical education discourse. *Academic Medicine: Journal of the Association of American Medical Colleges, 87*(9), 1185–1190. https://doi.org/10.1097/ACM.0b013e3182604968

30 Helmich, E., Yeh, H. M., Yeh, C. C., de Vries, J., Fu-Chang Tsai, D., & Dornan, T. (2017). Emotional learning and identity development in medicine: A cross-cultural qualitative study comparing Taiwanese and Dutch medical undergraduates. *Academic Medicine: Journal of the Association of American Medical Colleges, 92*(6), 853–859. https://doi.org/10.1097/ACM.0000000000001658

31 Elton, C. (2019). *Also human: The inner lives of doctors.* Windmill Books.

work.[32,33,34] Several authors are concerned that professional training consumes mental and affective resources, resulting in stunted development in the early years of the physician journey. **Kern** et al. assert that physician personal growth is promoted by "powerful experiences, helping relationships, and introspection," which lead to "changes in values, goals, or direction; healthier behaviors; improved connectedness with others; improved sense of self; and increased productivity, energy, or creativity."[35] **Horowitz** et al. write that what doctors find meaningful about their work includes instances of "a fundamental change in the doctor's perspective, a connection with patients, and a difference made in someone's life." They add, "transformational experiences … expanded the boundaries of their role as scientifically detached observers and prescribers of tests and treatments. They recognized their patients as fellow human beings, rather than objects of care."

In addition, **Halpern** finds addressing physician detachment and failures of emotional engagement in the formative years to be of utmost importance, an observation seconded by **Pu** et al. in a study of pediatric residents investigating the development of humanism and meaning in their training.

Stress is a constant presence on the journey to becoming a physician, with burnout, impairment, disillusionment, and threats to doctors' health imminent throughout their trajectory.[36,37] **Dyrbye** et al. describe levels of burnout and dissatisfaction among US physicians by life cycle stages, reporting:

32 Horowitz, C. R., Suchman, A. L., Branch, W. T., & Frankel, R. M. (2003). What do doctors find meaningful about their work? *Annals of Internal Medicine, 138*(9), 772–775. https://doi.org/10.7326/0003-4819-138-9-200305060-00028

33 Halpern, J. (2014). From idealized clinical empathy to empathic communication in medical care. *Medicine, Health Care, and Philosophy, 17*(2), 301–311. https://doi.org/10.1007/s11019-013-9510-4

34 Pu, H., Bachrach, L. K., & Blankenburg, R. (2022). Finding meaning in medicine: Pediatric residents' perspectives on humanism. *Academic Pediatrics, 22*(4), 680–688. https://doi.org/10.1016/j.acap.2021.12.007

35 Kern, D. E., Wright, S. M., Carrese, J. A., Lipkin, M. Jr., Simmons, J. M., Novack, D. H., Kalet, A., & Frankel, R. (2001). Personal growth in medical faculty: A qualitative study. *Western Journal of Medicine, 175*(2), 92–98. https://doi.org/10.1136/ewjm.175.2.92

36 Horton, J. (2021). *We are all perfectly fine: A memoir of love, medicine and healing.* HarperCollins.

37 Melnick, E. R., Dyrbye, L. N., Sinsky, C. A., Trockel, M., West, C. P., Nedelec, L., Tutty, M. A., & Shanafelt, T. (2020). The association between perceived electronic health record usability and professional burnout among US physicians. *Mayo Clinic Proceedings, 95*(3), 476–487. https://doi.org/10.1016/j.mayocp.2019.09.024

Early career physicians had the lowest satisfaction with overall career choice (being a physician), the highest frequency of work-home conflicts, and the highest rates of depersonalization (all *P*<.001). Physicians in middle career worked more hours, took more overnight calls, had the lowest satisfaction with their specialty choice and their work-life balance, and had the highest rates of emotional exhaustion and burnout (all *P*<.001). Middle career physicians were most likely to plan to leave the practice of medicine for reasons other than retirement in the next 24 months (4.8%, 12.5%, and 5.2% for early, middle, and late career, respectively). The challenges of middle career were observed in both men and women and across specialties and practice types.[38]

Thus, developmentally, emergent and established physicians are continuously oscillating between two poles. The first is positive and integrative, marked by expansion and growth, and features positive involvement in everyday practices and productive personal reflection. The second is disruptive and disabling, with arrests in development, potential ensuing impairment, and sometimes abandonment of the profession. Reports on the full impact of the coronavirus pandemic on this oscillation are forthcoming.[39,40]

RITES OF PASSAGE AND LIMINALITY

The physician's trajectory also features **passages**. These are nodes with qualitative differences in ways of knowing and transitions that elicit strong **feelings of defensiveness and vulnerability** in the learner. At these transitional points, too, self-efficacy may grow or diminish, and a sense of control over one's life and career may ebb or flow (see also Chapter 6). There is growing recognition of **learning moments, critical events, and**

38 Dyrbye, L. N., Varkey, P., Boone, S. L., Satele, D. V., Sloan, J. A., & Shanafelt, T. D. (2013). Physician satisfaction and burnout at different career stages. *Mayo Clinic Proceedings*, *88*(12), 1358–1367. https://doi.org/10.1016/j.mayocp.2013.07.016

39 Jalili, M., Niroomand, M., Hadavand, F., Zeinali, K., & Fotouhi, A. (2021). Burnout among healthcare professionals during COVID-19 pandemic: A cross-sectional study. *International Archives of Occupational and Environmental Health*, *94*(6), 1345–1352. https://doi.org/10.1007/s00420-021-01695-x

40 Rowe, S. G., Stewart, M. T., Van Horne, S., Pierre, C., Wang, H., Manukyan, M., Bair-Merritt, M., Lee-Parritz, A., Rowe, M. P., Shanafelt, T., & Trockel, M. (2022). Mistreatment experiences, protective workplace systems, and occupational distress in physicians. *JAMA Network Open*, *5*(5), e2210768. https://doi.org/10.1001/jamanetworkopen.2022.10768

obligatory rites of passage that carry with them possible breakthroughs and turning points as well as losses and corruption of development.

Van Gennep and **Turner** expand upon the perspective that the physician life cycle is comprised of multiple transitions, introducing the constructs of **rites of passage and liminality** (borrowed from anthropology) to the life cycle discourse.[41,42,43,44] Recently, **Gordon** et al. further contributed to this discussion by studying recorded transition diaries of United Kingdom proto-consultants.[45,46] In the preclinical years, cadaver dissection is a universal rite of passage[47,48] (albeit now becoming a thing of the past in many schools), and frequent transitioning from one clerkship to another is accompanied by rites of passage such as the first death of a patient, first intimate examination, and first delivery of a baby. Further transitions take place during internship and residency via clinical exposures, increased responsibility, and role and identity changes. Down the road, in midlife, comes the initial phase of practice as a specialist, with optional diversification of roles, followed by the transition to late career and retirement. The interplay of the biological life cycle and gender (pregnancy and the fertility age window for women), the relationships/ family life cycle, and the professional life cycle create incessant points of transition, conflict, uncertainty, and liminality.

Some rites of passage are formal: graduations and certifications (MD and specialist); assuming clinical, administrative, and academic roles;

41 Watts, T. E. (2013). Big ideas: 'Les rites de passage' Arnold van Gennep 1909. *Nurse Education Today*, *33*(4), 312–313. https://doi.org/10.1016/j.nedt.2012.09.010

42 Callaghan, A., Wearn, A., & Barrow, M. (2019). Providing a liminal space: Threshold concepts for learning in palliative medicine. *Medical Teacher*, *42*(4), 1–7. https://doi .org/10.1080/0142159X.2019.1687868

43 Browne, J. (2019). Living comfortably in liminal spaces: Trickster and the medical educator. *Medical Education*, *53*(1), 6–8. https://doi.org/10.1111/medu.13753

44 Janusz, B., & Walkiewicz, M. (2018). The rites of passage framework as a matrix of transgression processes in the life course. *Journal of Adult Development*, *25*(3), 151–159. https://doi.org/10.1007/s10804-018-9285-1

45 Gordon, L., Rees, C. E., & Jindal-Snape, D. (2020). Doctors' identity transitions: Choosing to occupy a state of 'betwixt and between'. *Medical Education*, *54*(11), 1006–1018. https://doi.org/10.1111/medu.14219

46 Gordon, L., Teunissen, P. W., Jindal-Snape, D., Bates, J., Rees, C. E., Westerman, M., Sinha, R., & van Dijk, A. (2020). An international study of trainee-trained transitions: Introducing the transition-to-trained-doctor (T3D) model. *Medical Teacher*, *42*(6), 679–688. https://doi.org/10.1080/0142159X.2020.1733508

47 Warner, J. H., & Rizzolo, L. J. (2006). Anatomical instruction and training for professionalism from the 19th to the 21st centuries. *Clinical Anatomy*, *19*(5), 403–414. https://doi.org/10.1002/ca.20290

48 Swick, H. M. (2006). Medical professionalism and the clinical anatomist. *Clinical Anatomy*, *19*(5), 393–402. https://doi.org/10.1002/ca.20258

climbing the academic rank ladder; continuously attempting to expand one's CV; and many others that are more tacit.[49]

Liminality is defined as "the psychological process of transitioning across boundaries and borders."[50] Introducing a structural aspect to the concept, van Gennep describes a three-stage liminality sequence: separation, transition, and incorporation. The first phase, "separation," refers to leaving the previous state or to the loss of a position achieved in life. The middle phase, "transition," also called the "liminal phase," is the crisis phase, characterized by uncertainty, disruption of order, and suspension of an important social structure. "Incorporation," the third phase, entails a new social identity and marks the start of a new period of life.

By studying liminality and identity in United Kingdom physicians transitioning to the role of consultant, Gordon et al. have contributed further insights, vocabulary, and a deeper elucidation of the inner work done by evolving medical practitioners. They report:

> We explored liminal experiences narrated by doctors across trainee-trained transitions. … Participants experienced liminality in three ways. First, most experienced temporary liminality at some point. Through identity work, participants engaged in self-reflection and considered past, present and future selves in order to expedite shifts towards this [sic] or her new identity, often relying on "consultant" identity grants from others to move them out of liminality. Second, … some doctors experienced perpetual liminality, undergoing enduring in-betweenness through dual roles. Participants were seen to use identity work to make themselves contextually and socially relevant, becoming boundary bricoleurs responding to competing loyalties and demands by continuously switching identities (e.g., from clinician to academic). Third, and novel to theoretical notions of liminality, individuals would sometimes purposely occupy liminality through its active creation and maintenance. … We suggest that … individuals can and do actively choose to be liminars, thereby exerting agency and control over his or her own liminality. … Our analysis revealed that a conceptualization of liminality as a linear progression from one professional identity (e.g., trainee doctor) to another (e.g.,

---

49 Teunissen, P. W., & Westerman, M. (2011). Opportunity or threat: The ambiguity of the consequences of transitions in medical education. *Medical Education*, 45(1), 51–59. https://doi.org/10.1111/j.1365-2923.2010.03755.x

50 Larson, P. (2014). Liminality. In D. A. Leeming (Ed.), *Encyclopedia of psychology and religion*. Springer. https://doi.org/10.1007/978-1-4614-6086-2_387

trained doctor) is overly simplistic. Indeed, through our temporal analysis of individuals' experiences across the longitudinal dataset, we noted that participants did not always proceed in a linear manner through the liminal phase.

Reflecting on these constructs suggests the multiplicity of liminal nodes in the doctor's life cycle (DLC): the professional transitions and rites of passage; personal stages of late adolescence, early and late adulthood, and old age; and building intimacy, relationships, and family, as well as entering parenthood, while also being a member of one's family of origin and participating in its transitions and crises. Thus, the practitioner likely experiences separation, suspension, and incorporation almost incessantly while dealing with at least one aspect of the life trajectory and often several. We return to the work of Gordon et al. in Chapter 9, where their findings on identity work seem most appropriate.

CRITICS OF STAGE MODELS, AND ONE DOCTOR'S REFLECTIONS ON DEVELOPMENTAL STAGES

Critics of the stage model paradigm have emerged in the last two decades. **Dall'Alba** argues that stage models ignore the embodied understanding of practice, which is dynamic, intersubjective, and pluralistic.[51] Thus, within a specific stage, multiple embodiment trajectories are possible and may even be contradictory. Dall'Alba's critique is further elaborated upon in Chapters 3 and 9.[52] Also, Bleakley et al. assert that the stage model is strikingly individual and ignores development as a social act that involves a community of practice (see Chapter 2).

Ventres provides a succinct example of a personal reflection on physician developmental stages. He summarizes his life cycle of doctoring, identifying his stages of developmental growth: competence, capability, responsibility, capacity, and citizenship (Figure 1.2). Similarly to Berger, Kleinman, and Morland, he adds a more personal lens to his report by incorporating representative concerns of "hope" and "worry" at each stage. Ventres concludes:

---

51 Dall'Alba, G., & Sandberg, J. (2006). Unveiling professional development: A critical review of stage models. *Review of Educational Research*, 76(3), 383–412. https://doi.org/10.3102/00346543076003383

52 Lee, J. H. (2017). The weaponization of medical professionalism. *Academic Medicine: Journal of the Association of American Medical Colleges*, 92(5), 579–580. https://doi.org/10.1097/ACM.0000000000001647

Developmental Period		Stage of Professional Growth	Representative Concerns	
			Hope	**Worry**
Medical school	Preclinical	Competence	Would I pass with honors?	Would I just "sneak by" or even fail?
	Clinical		Would I be recognized for my knowledge?	Could I hide my not knowing?
Residency	PGY-1		Would I save someone's life?	Would I cause someone's death?
	PGY-2/PGY-3		Would I be recognized for my competence?	Would I be blamed for some untoward patient outcome?
Early practice		Capability	Would patients see me as their physician?	Would I make a big mistake?
Middle practice		Responsibility	Could I grow my practice in scope and depth?	Would I stagnate in the routine?
Early mature practice		Capacity	Could I adapt in light of ongoing changes to medical practice?[a]	Would these changes obscure the humanistic aspects of medicine?[a]
Late mature practice[b]		Citizenship	Can I communicate the worth of a relational practice to others?[7,8]	Will the relational practice of medicine disappear in the face of ignorance and misunderstanding?[15]
Future practice		?	?	?

Abbreviation: PGY, postgraduate year.

[a] Changes to medical practice include desktop medicine, examination room computers, and system-based measures of quality.
[b] Late mature practice: the author's current level of professional development.

FIGURE 1.2 Developmental Periods, Stages of Professional Growth, and Example Concerns (Reproduced with permission from *JGME*. Ventres, W. B. 2014. Becoming a doctor: One physician's journey beyond competence. *Journal of Graduate Medical Education*, 6(4), 631–633. https://doi.org/10.4300/JGME-D-14-00144.1.)

> In sharing this snippet of my history, I hope that we … at the same time both use, and look beyond, competencies, milestones, and entrustable professional activities as measures of professional maturity. As we check a requisite box, may we remember the progress of our own advancement. As we fill in a standardized evaluation, may we recall the meaningful events that have sustained us in our practice and teaching roles. As we plan a curriculum, may we encourage our students and residents to reflect on their own professional growth. Only then, can we visualize as our overriding objective the much more expansive and ongoing process of becoming a physician and help those in our tutelage along their personal paths toward that goal.

In conclusion, following the prevalent developmental stage model movement in the second half of the 20th century, a developmental discourse ensued. Initially rooted in a psychodynamic orientation, it subsequently took on a cognitive psychology twist and then diversified to include additional theories, issues, and approaches, with professional identity formation as the most salient one. While a unifying theory or model has yet to emerge, stages are prominent. First, lifespan developmental stages; subsequently, professional career and identity developmental stages, later expanded upon with the subcategorical aspects of career, expertise, character, reflective practice, morality, and leadership. The critical nature of transitions between stages and roles, formal and informal, is highlighted. Tasks, passages, conflicts, and polarizations are described. Many constructs emerge, including cognition, emotion, and metacognition; self-representations (identities) that extend beyond knowledge, attitudes, and skills; engagement and disengagement (empathy and detachment); the conflict of vulnerability versus omnipotence; boundary management; agency and control issues; and, finally, liminality and identity work. These are further discussed in the upcoming categories. Kegan's theory stands out, lasting for more than four decades and gradually making inroads into medical education.

Summary

As early as 1957, Merton postulates the basic ingredients of becoming a physician: knowledge, skills, feeling like a physician, and assuming the physician's identity. Subsequently, multiple scholars describe stages of personal and professional development, initially with a psychodynamic approach and later introducing additional perspectives. Kegan stands out by suggesting a robust theory of development that is associated with assessment, which most other approaches lack. His framework is later applied in various additional subcategories. Furthermore, the concept of liminality, which sheds light on transitions in the DLC, is introduced. An example of one practitioner's reflections and personal review of his development is provided. Critics of the stage model highlight its linear, reductionist nature and, as of late, question its overlooking issues of inclusivity as well as the impact of the coronavirus pandemic. Many of these aspects find an echo in the narratives opening the chapters of this book. This category sets the stage for the upcoming categories and may find its ultimate place in PIF (Chapter 9).

REFERENCES

Becker, H., Geer, B., Hughes, E. C., & Strauss, A. L. (1976). *Boys in white: Student culture in medical school* (Reprint ed.). Transaction Publishers.

Berger, J. G. (2002). A summary of the constructive-developmental theory of Robert Kegan.

Brent, D. A. (1981). The residency as a developmental process. *Journal of Medical Education*, 56(5), 417–422. https://doi.org/10.1097/00001888-198105000-00006

Browne, J. (2019). Living comfortably in liminal spaces: Trickster and the medical educator. *Medical Education*, 53(1), 6–8. https://doi.org/10.1111/medu.13753

Callaghan, A., Wearn, A., & Barrow, M. (2019). Providing a liminal space: Threshold concepts for learning in palliative medicine. *Medical Teacher*, 42(4), 1–7. https://doi.org/10.1080/0142159X.2019.1687868

Carroll, J. G., Lipkin, M., Nachtigall, L., & Weston, W. W. (1995). A developmental awareness for teaching doctor/patient communication skills. In M. Lipkin, S. M. Putnam, A. Lazare, J. G. Carroll, & R. M., Frankel (Eds.), *The medical interview* (pp. 388–396). Frontiers of Primary Care. Springer. https://doi.org/10.1007/978-1-4612-2488-4_32

Dall'Alba, G., & Sandberg, J. (2006). Unveiling professional development: A critical review of stage models. *Review of Educational Research*, 76(3), 383–412. https://doi.org/10.3102/00346543076003383

Davis, B., & Francis, K. (2021). Discourses on learning in education: Making sense of a landscape of difference. *Frontiers in Education*, 6, 1–12.

Dyrbye, L. N., Varkey, P., Boone, S. L., Satele, D. V., Sloan, J. A., & Shanafelt, T. D. (2013). Physician satisfaction and burnout at different career stages. *Mayo Clinic Proceedings*, 88(12), 1358–1367. https://doi.org/10.1016/j.mayocp.2013.07.016

Elton, C. (2019). *Also human: The inner lives of doctors*. Windmill Books.

Erikson, E. H. (1968). *Identity, youth and crisis*. W.W. Norton Company.

Erikson, E. H. (1976). Reflections on Dr. Borg's life cycle. *Daedalus*, 105(2), 1–28.

Forsythe, G. B. (2005). Identity development in professional education. *Academic Medicine: Journal of the Association of American Medical Colleges*, 80(Suppl 10), S112–S117. https://doi.org/10.1097/00001888-200510001-00029

Forsythe, G. B., Snook, S., Lewis, P., & Bartone, P. T. (2002). Making sense of officership: Developing a professional identity for 21st century army officers. In D. M. Snider & G. L. Watkins (Eds.), *The future of the army profession* (pp. 357–378). McGraw-Hill.

General Medical Council. (2018). *Outcomes for graduates*. https://www.gmc-uk.org/-/media/documents/dc11326-outcomes-for-graduates-2018_pdf-75040796.pdf

Gordon, L., Rees, C. E., & Jindal-Snape, D. (2020). Doctors' identity transitions: Choosing to occupy a state of 'betwixt and between'. *Medical Education, 54*(11), 1006–1018. https://doi.org/10.1111/medu.14219

Gordon, L., Teunissen, P. W., Jindal-Snape, D., Bates, J., Rees, C. E., Westerman, M., Sinha, R., & van Dijk, A. (2020). An international study of trainee-trained transitions: Introducing the transition-to-trained-doctor (T3D) model. *Medical Teacher, 42*(6), 679–688. https://doi.org/10.1080/0142159X.2020.1733508

Halpern, J. (2014). From idealized clinical empathy to empathic communication in medical care. *Medicine, Health Care, and Philosophy, 17*(2), 301–311. https://doi.org/10.1007/s11019-013-9510-4

Helmich, E., Yeh, H. M., Yeh, C. C., de Vries, J., Fu-Chang Tsai, D., & Dornan, T. (2017). Emotional learning and identity development in medicine: A cross-cultural qualitative study comparing Taiwanese and Dutch medical undergraduates. *Academic Medicine: Journal of the Association of American Medical Colleges, 92*(6), 853–859. https://doi.org/10.1097/ACM.0000000000001658

Horowitz, C. R., Suchman, A. L., Branch, W. T., & Frankel, R. M. (2003). What do doctors find meaningful about their work? *Annals of Internal Medicine, 138*(9), 772–775. https://doi.org/10.7326/0003-4819-138-9-200305060-00028

Horton, J. (2021). *We are all perfectly fine: A memoir of love, medicine and healing.* HarperCollins.

Jalili, M., Niroomand, M., Hadavand, F., Zeinali, K., & Fotouhi, A. (2021). Burnout among healthcare professionals during COVID-19 pandemic: A cross-sectional study. *International Archives of Occupational and Environmental Health, 94*(6), 1345–1352. https://doi.org/10.1007/s00420-021-01695-x

Janusz, B., & Walkiewicz, M. (2018). The rites of passage framework as a matrix of transgression processes in the life course. *Journal of Adult Development, 25*(3), 151–159. https://doi.org/10.1007/s10804-018-9285-1

Jarvis-Selinger, S., Pratt, D. D., & Regehr, G. (2012). Competency is not enough: Integrating identity formation into the medical education discourse. *Academic Medicine: Journal of the Association of American Medical Colleges, 87*(9), 1185–1190. https://doi.org/10.1097/ACM.0b013e3182604968

Kalet, A., Ark, T. K., Monson, V., Song, H. S., Buckvar-Keltz, L., Harnik, V., Yingling, S., Rivera, R., Jr, Tewksbury, L., Lusk, P., & Crowe, R. (2021). Does a measure of medical professional identity formation predict communication skills performance? *Patient Education and Counseling, 104*(12), 3045–3052. https://doi.org/10.1016/j.pec.2021.03.040

Kegan, R. (2009). What "form" transforms? A constructive-developmental approach to transformative learning. In K. Illeris (Ed.), *Contemporary theories of learning: Learning theorists in their own words* (pp 35–54). Routledge.

Kern, D. E., Wright, S. M., Carrese, J. A., Lipkin, M. Jr., Simmons, J. M., Novack, D. H., Kalet, A., & Frankel, R. (2001). Personal growth in medical faculty: A qualitative study. *Western Journal of Medicine, 175*(2), 92–98. https://doi.org/10.1136/ewjm.175.2.92

Larson, P. (2014). Liminality. In D. A. Leeming (Ed.), *Encyclopedia of psychology and Religion.* Springer. https://doi.org/10.1007/978-1-4614-6086-2_387

Lee, J. H. (2017). The weaponization of medical professionalism. *Academic Medicine: Journal of the Association of American Medical Colleges, 92*(5), 579–580. https://doi.org/10.1097/ACM.0000000000001647

Levinson, D. J. (1967). Medical education and the theory of adult socialization. *Journal of Health and Social Behavior, 8*(4), 253–265. https://psycnet.apa.org/doi/10.2307/2948419

Levinson, D. J. (1980). Toward a conception of the adult life course. In N. J. Smelser (Ed.), *Themes of work and love in adulthood.* Harvard University Press.

Lewin, L. O., McManamon, A., Stein, M. T. O., & Chen, D. T. (2019). Minding the form that transforms: Using Kegan's model of adult development to understand personal and professional identity formation in medicine. *Academic Medicine: Journal of the Association of American Medical Colleges*, 94(9), 1299–1304. https://doi.org/10.1097/ACM.0000000000002741

Marcus, E. R. (1999). Empathy, humanism, and the professionalization process of medical education. *Academic Medicine: Journal of the Association of American Medical Colleges*, 74(11), 1211–1215. https://doi.org/10.1097/00001888-199911000-00014

Marcus, E. R. (2003). Medical student dreams about medical school: The unconscious developmental process of becoming a physician. *International Journal of Psycho-Analysis*, 84(Pt 2), 367–386. https://doi.org/10.1516/002075703321632964

Marcus, E. R. (2013). Wild strawberries. *Bulletin of the Association for Psychoanalytic Medicine*. Reproduced with permission of the author, 44.

Melnick, E. R., Dyrbye, L. N., Sinsky, C. A., Trockel, M., West, C. P., Nedelec, L., Tutty, M. A., & Shanafelt, T. (2020). The association between perceived electronic health record usability and professional burnout among US physicians. *Mayo Clinic Proceedings*, 95(3), 476–487. https://doi.org/10.1016/j.mayocp.2019.09.024

Merton, R. K., Reader, G. G., & Kendall, P. L. (Eds.). (1957). *The student physician: Introductory studies in the sociology of medical education*. Harvard University Press. http://dx.doi.org/10.4159/harvard.9780674366831

Pu, H., Bachrach, L. K., & Blankenburg, R. (2022). Finding meaning in medicine: Pediatric residents' perspectives on humanism. *Academic Pediatrics*, 22(4), 680–688. https://doi.org/10.1016/j.acap.2021.12.007

Quirk, M. (2006). *Intuition and metacognition in medical education: Keys to developing expertise*. Springer.

Roberts, L. W. (2020). Women and academic medicine, 2020. *Academic Medicine: Journal of the Association of American Medical Colleges*, 95(10), 1459–1464. https://doi.org/10.1097/ACM.0000000000003617

Rowe, S. G., Stewart, M. T., Van Horne, S., Pierre, C., Wang, H., Manukyan, M., Bair-Merritt, M., Lee-Parritz, A., Rowe, M. P., Shanafelt, T., & Trockel, M. (2022). Mistreatment experiences, protective workplace systems, and occupational distress in physicians. *JAMA Network Open*, 5(5), e2210768. https://doi.org/10.1001/jamanetworkopen.2022.10768

Rule, J. T., & Bebeau, M. J. (2005). *Dentists who care: Inspiring stories of professional commitment*. Quintessence Books.

Sheehy, G. (2006). *Passages: Predictable crises in adult life* (30th Anniversary ed.). Ballantine Books.

Swick, H. M. (2006). Medical professionalism and the clinical anatomist. *Clinical Anatomy*, 19(5), 393–402. https://doi.org/10.1002/ca.20258

Teunissen, P. W., & Westerman, M. (2011). Opportunity or threat: The ambiguity of the consequences of transitions in medical education. *Medical Education*, 45(1), 51–59. https://doi.org/10.1111/j.1365-2923.2010.03755.x

Ventres, W. B. (2014). Becoming a doctor: One physician's journey beyond competence. *Journal of Graduate Medical Education*, 6(4), 631–633. https://doi.org/10.4300/JGME-D-14-00144.1

Warner, J. H., & Rizzolo, L. J. (2006). Anatomical instruction and training for professionalism from the 19th to the 21st centuries. *Clinical Anatomy*, 19(5), 403–414. https://doi.org/10.1002/ca.20290

Watts, T. E. (2013). Big ideas: 'Les rites de passage' Arnold van Gennep 1909. *Nurse Education Today*, 33(4), 312–313. https://doi.org/10.1016/j.nedt.2012.09.010

Weston, W. W., & Brown, J. B. (2024). Becoming a physician: The human experience of medical education. In M. Stewart, J. B. Brown, W. W. Weston, T. R. Freeman, B. L. Ryan, C. L. McWilliam, & I. R. McWhinney (Eds.), *Patient-centered medicine: Transforming the clinical method* (4th ed.). CRC Press.

Weston, W. W., & Lipkin, M. Jr. (1989). Doctors learning communication skill: Developmental issues. In M. Stewart & D. Roter (Eds.), *Communicating with medical patients* (pp. 43–57). Sage Publications.

Zabarenko, R. N., & Zabarenko, L. M. (1978). *The doctor tree: Developmental stages in the growth of physicians.* University of Pittsburgh Press.

Zabarenko, R. N., Zabarenko, L., & Pittenger, R. A. (1970). The psychodynamics of physicianhood. *Psychiatry, 33*(1), 102–118. https://doi.org/10.1080/00332747.1970.11023617

CHAPTER 2

Adult learning and continuous medical education

The practice years

....

Learning through vulnerability: A mentor–mentee experience

At the start of my third year of family medicine training, I began to fear that I was falling off the normal resident development curve as I struggled to fit my patients' complicated needs within an increasingly short clinic visit. … My residency director suggested I pilot a residency mentoring program with a visiting physician.

After almost 30 years of rural practice and academic work at the Technion in Haifa, Israel, I finally took a year-long sabbatical. … One of the first ideas that came up in discussion with the department chair was to work with the residents. He devised a title: Advanced Clinical Mentoring. I liked the idea, yet I had no idea how it would unfold. Yes, this prospect was risky, and I was anxious, outside my language, away from my home environment, preparing to step into the role of advanced clinician, whatever that meant.

We met in the morning just before your clinic. You told me what you were hoping to accomplish—managing time and reenergizing your morale for the task beyond residency. … There was a student as well. … We jumped in.

We were three generations of physicians. As our entourage entered each examination room, … the patients smiled at the progression of learning, and we moved through our afternoon schedule.

DOI: 10.1201/9781003507529-3

So strange, I was a fly on the wall, doing nothing but noticing. … I observed for a few minutes, then reached into my pocket and took out my notebook. Taking notes helped keep my anxiety in check. I was writing notes intuitively: some clinical details and the rest observations and running commentary.

Would I make sense when it came to the actual mentoring?

The medical student described the first patient to me: "Thirty-three years old with a history of breast cysts with tenderness; she's afraid she has breast cancer."

"What's her family history?"

We returned to the room to find out.

She told us details of her pain, of her life, and revealed that, yes, her mom had breast cancer diagnosed at age 33, and died ten years later. She began to cry.

"I'm so worried I have cancer too."

I comforted her, counseled her, talked of mammograms, ultrasound procedures, and genetic counseling. Then I asked her to undress for the breast examination and left the room, where nurses accosted me with forms to sign for other patients, then my pager beeped with an urgent call about a patient in drug rehab, and suddenly 15 minutes had evaporated. I didn't realize it until the patient came into the hallway wrapped in her paper gown and demanded to know what was taking so long.

I had acknowledged her fears of cancer, and then left her alone with them naked in the examining room. … I decided to send her for the mammogram and ultrasonography without the breast examination and continued my day.

I witnessed your moment of difficulty; part of me was sinking in tandem. You took a long moment to collect yourself, then changed course. I wrote to myself: Critical incident, good decision making.

It clicks in for me. I am not a foreigner in the land of patients, their care, and docs, nor am I a stranger to deep listening and empathy. I navigate, putting myself in the patient's shoes, your shoes, and the student's shoes. I feel joy seeing how my years of practice and reflection become handy.

In our wrap-up discussion at the end of our first day together, I returned to this patient interaction, which demonstrates both what I love and hate about medicine. … I love treating not just symptoms, but addressing the psychosocial environment that makes those symptoms appear in the first place.

I hate keeping people waiting while I try to provide everything for everybody, in the process frustrating my patients, my staff, and myself.

At the end of the day, you wanted insight and empowerment for action. I was reactive, transmitting practical/technical models and ideas, such as family-orientation, Medalie's levels of practice,[1] agenda setting,[2] and the One-Minute

1   Medalie, J.H. (1978). Introduction. In Medalie, J.H. (Ed.), *Family medicine: Principles and applications.* Williams & Wilkins.

2   Freeman, T. (2016). *McWhinney's textbook of family medicine* (4th ed.). Oxford University Press.

Preceptor.[3] *... This was my first advanced clinical mentoring (whatever it meant), and it felt fragile and precious and risky, yet strangely familiar and liberating. By being attentive and mindful, accepting risk and vulnerability, we were creating a learning opportunity for both of us.*

You presented a solution. If I wanted to be able to go home at a reasonable time with no more charts to write, no lingering unreturned telephone calls, I'd need to learn how to limit my scope of practice.

I'd need to find out what they wanted from the visit and to shape the visit to meet their agenda. ... If I could widen my scope of practice for just one clinic visit each day, and go home happy, my day complete, I would have succeeded in becoming the family physician I dreamt of becoming.

You also introduced me to the concept of the One-Minute Preceptor, asking medical students to respond to pointed clinical questions. ... I could quickly assess medical students' level of knowledge and teach to their learning needs.

During our wrap-up, I modeled the One-Minute Preceptor, the clinical training tool for teaching on the fly about clinical problem solving, eliciting your reasoning (as well as needs) and commenting briefly. Here we adapt it to mentoring on the fly. Is it working? It seems so. I can relax a bit now.

After our session together, I consciously limited my scope of practice to the chief complaint before me that day. When patients tried to ask for more than we could address in our allotted time, I reminded them we had 15 minutes and asked them to choose what they wanted to deal with that day. Simple, no? I learned so much from the first session, I requested another mentoring session.

During the second session with you three weeks later, two tattooed men, two heel spurs, a breast lump, and then "Mr. 18 issues" (with many more in review of systems), a murderer. Your first murderer, I've seen a few, but nothing like that one. You already implemented the agenda setting we discussed: "What would you like me to do for you today?"

I saw an overweight woman complaining of pain from her heel spurs that ibuprofen wouldn't touch. ... She wanted controlled substances, I didn't want to give them, and we spent too long negotiating for her to end up with what she wanted anyway, with the caveat that there would be no refills without her trying physical therapy.

Ian McWhinney's patient-centered clinical method comes to mind: noticing the doctor's and patient's agendas and evaluating their concordance. It will not work, in spite of best intentions, to make a patient do physical therapy if she has a diametrically opposite agenda. It can save a lot of energy and frustration to diagnose

3   Neher, J. O., Gordon, K. C., Meyer, B., & Stevens, N. (1992). A five-step "microskills" model of clinical teaching. *Journal of the American Board of Family Practice*, 5(4), 419–424.

this mismatch. I point it out to you, and you are applying it in the next complex patient. What a joy!

And then there was Monsieur Manslaughterer.

"He's complicated," you said, my time watcher and encounter understander. "He presented 18 problems in 10 to 15 minutes."

Bipolar. Post-traumatic stress disorder. Homeless. Phoneless. Gay and unable to live with his lover because of housing regulations allowing spouses, but no roommates. Noncompliant with medications. Refusing to see a psychologist. He proudly showed off the scars on his arms that landed him in the psychiatric hospital last year for ten days. He wanted to talk about his tooth pain. And back pain. And joint pain. And full-body, full-life pain.

Not to mention a long former history of sexual abuse, restless legs syndrome, eye twitching, and a 21-year-old son who still comes back home to live there.

"I'm a pain in the ass!" he said, proudly.

He comes to us for Percocet, prescribed by the doctors of this clinic. But we can't medicate away a pain in the ass, the pain of his life—of his no-good, beaten-up, man-murdering life. Five years he spent in jail.

"He abused me, I stabbed him, he died."

After he mentioned his current suicidality, I delayed his routine care and handed him off to our staff psychologist, who knew him well. "He's been here before," she sighed, after going into the room with the patient and walking him to a phone to call his case manager. "I've done exactly this, not just once but twice before."

Impressive containment. Trust the clinic process. The system works.

Our mentoring is working too. We are moving fast from my observations to your empowered action with the next patients. You are no longer overwhelmed. Neither am I.

I am learning to trust the mentoring process. Our system works—authentically being present, using models that fit the situation to cognitively scaffold the learning, and identifying learning opportunities that transcend and integrate the problem solving.

By inviting a senior physician to observe my clinical encounters for an entire clinic session, encompassing both smooth and difficult patient interactions, I gained confidence in myself as a clinician. By opening myself to feedback and new learning models, I learned to be a more efficient doctor for difficult patients, and a more effective clinical teacher. …

From McWhinney, I have learned to determine the patient agenda, acknowledge that we can't do everything in a single visit, and together we prioritize their problems. …

When they expect too much, I say: "We have 15 minutes together today. You can come back in two weeks, and we'll give each problem the attention it deserves."

From Medalie, I have learned to recognize when a patient's needs are beyond a doctor–patient clinical encounter: "Let me put you in touch with my colleague."

I hand off the psychological needs to the psychologist, the social needs to the social worker. … I remain focused on addressing and ameliorating the physical symptoms, diagnosing, and treating disease in 15 minutes or less.

Applying the One-Minute Preceptor model, I have learned to elicit what medical students know and teach them what they have not yet learned.

"What do you think is going on? What do you want to do? Why?"

In very little time I acknowledge their strengths and teach to their weaknesses. Through my mentor, I have learned from the masters.

Learning from vulnerability is the construct that starts resonating with me—this is how I have grown, this is how you are growing now. In this mentoring experience I have been moving away from my comfort zone, pushing my safety limits. We all get uncomfortable as we reach our safety limits; we become vulnerable. By embracing this vulnerability, growth becomes possible. When I am mindful of my fear and at the same time notice, reflect on, and accept it, I may be breaking through my vulnerabilities to a position of strength. In this process, I extended what I am able to do comfortably.

We drew on direct clinical observation followed by the transmittance of clinic models from the mentor to the mentee as a springboard for clinical growth. I subsequently applied this ongoing process of learning to other residents, to senior faculty including the chair, and in other departments. Three months down the road I was shadowing a senior doc at a distant institution, and a year later I am introducing it at home.

All clinicians at all stages of training and mentoring are lifelong learners. Advanced Clinical Mentoring provides a model for the continuing medical education of clinical skills.[4]

* * *

Although the focus of this opening story is the clinical supervision of a resident, the inclusion of the mentor's inner dialogue provides a stream-of-consciousness account of a highly experienced physician taking on a risky role—one associated with vulnerability and liminality—that turns into a rewarding developmental experience.

---

4   Jones, K., & Reis, S. (2010). Learning through vulnerability: A mentor-mentee experience. *Annals of Family Medicine*, 8(6), 552–555. https://doi.org/10.1370/afm.1165. Reproduced with permission.

LIFELONG LEARNING AND CAREER STAGES

Springing initially from literature on continuous medical education (CME), and more recently from a wave of writing about "becoming a professional," another attempt at addressing the professional life cycle of physicians has emerged. This time, the discourse looks mostly at the third stage, the practice years. Developed, again, from basic studies in adult development and learning,[5,6,7,8] and initially focused on other disciplines such as education, business, theology, nursing, engineering, and the military,[9,10] the idea and empirical evidence showing that professionals grow and change throughout their careers, not only in the formal formative years, is in its nascence when it comes to the working years stage of personal and professional development (PPD, or sometimes continuous professional development [CPD], as CME is called in the United Kingdom).[11]

The distinguishing features of adult learning include learner independence, extensive prior knowledge, varied motivations and expectations, varied learning styles, an expected change of attitudes when acquiring new skills, a preference for experiential learning, internal motivation, and the crucial importance of feedback rather than tests. These principles have informed the transformation of medical education. Since the end of the 20th century, innovative pedagogies fostering **self-regulated learning** as a springboard for developing **lifelong learning**

5   Fox, R. D. (2003). Continuing professional education. In J. W. Guthrie (Ed.), *Encyclopedia of education* (2nd ed.). Macmillan Reference USA.

6   Super, D. E. (1957). *The psychology of careers*. Harper.

7   Sullivan, S. E. (1999). The changing nature of careers: A review and research agenda. *Journal of Management, 25*(3), 457–484. https://doi.org/10.1177/014920639902500308

8   Bennett, N. L., & Hotvedt, M. O. (1989). Stage of career. In R. D. Fox, P. E. Mazmanian, & R. W. Putnam (Eds.), *Changing and learning in the lives of physicians*. Praeger.

9   Hedlund, J., Forsythe, G. B., Horvath, J. A., Williams, W. M., Snook, S., & Sternberg, R. J. (2003). Identifying and assessing tacit knowledge: Understanding the practical intelligence of military leaders. *Leadership Quarterly, 14*(2), 117–140. https://doi.org/10.1016/S1048-9843(03)00006-7

10 Palmer, P. J. (2017). *The courage to teach: Exploring the inner landscape of a teacher's life*. John Wiley & Sons.

11 Löffler, C., Altiner, A., Blumenthal, S., Bruno, P., De Sutter, A., De Vos, B. J., Dinant, G. J., Duerden, M., Dunais, B., Egidi, G., Gibis, B., Melbye, H., Rouquier, F., Rosemann, T., Touboul-Lundgren, P., & Feldmeier, G. (2022). Challenges and opportunities for general practice specific CME in Europe—A narrative review of seven countries. *BMC Medical Education, 22*(1), 761. https://doi.org/10.1186/s12909-022-03832-7

competence have been introduced in basic medical education and gradu-ate medical education (GME), as well as in CME. These changes have recast the doctor's life cycle (DLC) through the inclusion, in many coun-tries, of recertification and professional development plans and audits, all with increased regulatory and bureaucratic pressures.[12] Coupled with the digital age and the ubiquity of burdensome electronic medi-cal records (EMRs), and further fueled by the coronavirus pandemic, an epidemic of physician burnout has been documented and is on the rise worldwide.[13] Attention has thus been drawn to issues of **resilience and burnout prevention** as added components of doctor formation and lifelong development.

Needs-based CME was the first result of this approach.[14] Portfolios became a new educational and professional development strategy, while personal and professional development plans are now required in some countries. A description of stages and transitions followed, this time mapping out years in practice and focus of career in very practical terms.[15,16,17] Initially described for family physicians, these models sup-port a conceptual framework for understanding career stages and transi-tions. Furthermore, they can also provide guidance regarding the needs and wants of physicians, as well as the learning opportunities that enable physician development.

The developmental processes and stages of a career in family medi-cine were used to create a foundation for a lifelong learning curriculum

12 Ballouk, R., Mansour, V., Dalziel, B., McDonald, J., & Hegazi, I. (2022). Medical students' self-regulation of learning in a blended learning environment: A systematic scoping review. *Medical Education Online*, 27(1), 2029336. https://doi.org/10.1080/10872981.2022.2029336

13 Ryan, A., Hickey, A., Harkin, D., Boland, F., Collins, M. E., & Doyle, F. (2023). Professional identity formation, professionalism, leadership and resilience (PILLAR) in medical students: Methodology and early results. *Journal of Medical Education and Curricular Development*, 10. https://doi.org/10.1177/23821205231198921

14 Cohen, R., Amiel, G. E., Tann, M., Shechter, A., Weingarten, M., & Reis, S. (2002). Performance assessment of community-based physicians: Evaluating the reliability and validity of a tool for determining CME needs. *Academic Medicine: Journal of the Association of American Medical Colleges*, 77(12 Pt 1), 1247–1254. https://doi.org/10.1097/00001888-200212000-00022

15 Merriam, S. B., & Baumgartner, L. M. (2020). *Learning in adulthood: A comprehen-sive guide* (4th ed.). Jossey-Bass.

16 Little, M., & Midtling, J. E. (2011). *Becoming a family physician*. (Softcover reprint of the original 1st ed. 1989). Springer.

17 Jones, W. A., Avant, R. F., Davis, N., Saultz, J., & Lyons, P. (2004). Task force report 3. Report of the task force on continuous personal, professional, and practice devel-opment in family medicine. *Annals of Family Medicine*, 2(Suppl 1), s65–s74. https://doi.org/10.1370/afm.136

focused on the growth and development of physicians' personal, professional, and practice systems. The five stages in the career of a family physician are initiated with **graduation from residency, followed by a skill-building stage, midcareer, a mature phase, and finally a late-career stage**. Again, this is a stage model built around practicalities rather than the development of the professional's self or her expertise, and it seems applicable to most specialties. The opening narrative of this chapter illustrates this model, pairing a senior resident in the clinical skill-building stage with a late-career practitioner who is further developing advanced mentoring skills.

Bickel unpacks the midcareer stage, identifying a midlife crisis for physicians, especially those with an academic career. She addresses "growth-promoting strategies that midcareer faculty can tailor to individual needs, including questions for personal reflection."[18] Further, she highlights the healthy nature of reexamining commitments at this career stage by considering what one values most (see Chapter 1). Bickel states that research on adult development and resilience confirms her assertions and observes that shifting attention from personal and professional constraints to modifiable aspects of oneself and one's situation is key to further growth in midcareer.

The study of physician professional development toward the end of the 20th century introduced additional theoretical perspectives on learning. Situated learning and communities of practice, first proposed by **Lave** and **Wenger**,[19,20,21] both fall under the constructivist paradigm and emphasize learning in the workplace. Indeed, most of the doctor's trajectory will take place in the workplace. In addition, even in the preclinical years of BME, early exposure to the workplace, often in the community, is happening much more frequently. In situated learning, the key components are **cognitive apprenticeship, collaborative learning, reflection, deliberate practice** (see Chapter 3), and articulation of learning skills. **Community of practice** points out the process by which novice physicians move from the periphery of the community to eventually becoming fully integrated in it, and during this time they are shaped and molded in multiple informal ways.

---

18 Bickel, J. (2016). Not too late to reinvigorate: How midcareer faculty can continue growing. *Academic Medicine: Journal of the Association of American Medical Colleges*, 91(12), 1601–1605. https://doi.org/10.1097/ACM.0000000000001310

19 Lave, J., & Wenger, E. (1991). *Situated learning: Legitimate peripheral participation*. Cambridge University Press.

20 Wenger, E. (1998). *Communities of practice: Learning, meaning, and identity*. Cambridge University Press. https://doi.org/10.1017/CBO9780511803932

21 Le May, A. (2009). *Communities of practice in health and social care*. Wiley-Blackwell.

LIFELONG LEARNING PEDAGOGIES: CLINICAL SUPERVISION, MENTORING, AND SUPPORT

Launer introduced the notion of clinical supervision as a PPD mechanism.[22,23] He notes that **while knowledge accumulates, performance needs to be maintained**. Clinical supervision differs from formal learning, being a gradual, personal apprenticeship that helps the steady adjustment of competence through life.[24] He applies the term "conversations inviting change" to his method, adding questioning on top of listening to a narrative approach. This too is vividly present in this chapter's opening narrative.

Role modeling, mentoring, and coaching are additional pedagogies recently acknowledged as effective means for personal and professional development.[25,26] **Peer supervision, quality circles, and support groups** have become prevalent and support the need for "high touch" in the present "high tech" reality.[27] **Rabow** et al. state:

> To meet the complex medical and social challenges of the next century, medical educators must continue to promote cognitive expertise while *concurrently* supporting "professional formation" – the moral and professional development of students, their ability to stay true to their personal service values and the core values of the profession, and the integration of their individual maturation with growth in clinical competency.[28]

22 Burton, J., & Launer, J. (Eds.). (2003). *Supervision and support in primary care.* CRC Press.

23 Launer, J. (2019). Supervision, mentoring and coaching. In T. Swanwick, K. Forrest, & B. C. O'Brien (Eds.), *Understanding medical education—Evidence, theory, and practice* (pp. 179–190). John Wiley & Sons.

24 Launer, J. (2007). Moving on from Balint: Embracing clinical supervision. *British Journal of General Practice: The Journal of the Royal College of General Practitioners*, 57(536), 182–183.

25 Lovell, B. (2018). What do we know about coaching in medical education? A literature review. *Medical Education*, 52(4), 376–390. https://doi.org/10.1111/medu .13482

26 Foster, K., & Roberts, C. (2016). The heroic and the villainous: A qualitative study characterising the role models that shaped senior doctors' professional identity. *BMC Medical Education*, 16(1), 206. https://doi.org/10.1186/s12909-016-0731-0

27 Dehning, S., Reiß, E., Krause, D., Gasperi, S., Meyer, S., Dargel, S., Müller, N., & Siebeck, M. (2014). Empathy in high-tech and high-touch medicine. *Patient Education and Counseling*, 95(2), 259–264. https://doi.org/10.1016/j.pec.2014.01 .013

28 Rabow, M. W., Remen, R. N., Parmelee, D. X., & Inui, T. S. (2010). Professional formation: Extending medicine's lineage of service into the next century. *Academic Medicine: Journal of the Association of American Medical Colleges*, 85(2), 310–317. https://doi.org/10.1097/ACM.0b013e3181c887f7

PROFESSIONAL FORMATION

Foster et al.[29] echo the construct of **professional formation** in the education of clergy, later applied by **Benner** in nurse education,[30] connoting that the emerging professional is more than just a technical craftsperson, but rather a transformed person with the vocation or "calling" for healing.

Introducing professional identity formation (PIF) to adult learning and the CME years, **Lockyer** et al. assert that "while the formation of professional identity may be considered a phenomenon that occurs primarily during formal periods of learning, people do change over a career."[31] They introduce the notion that the DLC was radically different for the female physician due to the prevailing social roles women had in the past. The identity of "mother" was accompanied by an additional struggle for balancing life and work. Although these norms are changing, this experience remains more prevalent for female physicians. Moreover, studies are increasingly documenting adverse fertility outcomes, agonizing decisions concerning parenting and related stress, especially experienced by female students and residents. One result, among others, is that an evolving female practitioner has less free time for learning when children are added to the mix, as the rearing responsibility disproportionately falls on her.

The practice years are characterized by optional transitions in workplace, specialty, and often geographic location, with the stresses that these entail. These changes also offer opportunities for rapid professional and personal development. Navigating each new transition—getting in, fitting in, and getting out—demands specific attention and is taxing with regard to identity formation. Many settle into an independent practice, which is often more stable but fraught with additional transitions of focus, role, and community of practice. Identities that may be juggled in these circumstances include clinician, educator, researcher, and administrator, to name the salient ones. The next stage, that of transitioning out of practice and/or retiring, is another challenge to personal and professional identity. Other phenomena that influence identity during the practice years include teams, context, and specialization.

---

29 Foster, C. R., Dahill, L., Goleman, L. A., & Tolentino, B. W. (2005). *Educating clergy: Teaching practices and pastoral imagination.* Jossey-Bass.

30 Benner, P., Sutphen, M., Leonard-Kahn, V., & Day, L. (2008). Formation and everyday ethical comportment. *American Journal of Critical Care: An Official Publication, American Association of Critical-Care Nurses, 17*(5), 473–476.

31 Lockyer, J., de Groot, J., & Silver, I. (2016). Professional identity formation, the practicing physician and continuing professional development. In R. L. Cruess, S. R. Cruess, & Y. Steinert (Eds.), *Teaching medical professionalism: Supporting the development of a professional identity* (pp. 186–200). Cambridge University Press.

CURRENT APPROACHES TO PHYSICIAN
LIFELONG LEARNING

In the last decade, the discourse on adult learning and CME has grown more sophisticated. **Mazmanian** et al. suggest "an ecological framework" for "reimagining physician development and lifelong learning," which "advances a biopsychosocial viewpoint, emphasizing human agency and the value of age-graded events, roles, transitions, interaction, and heritability."[32] Their framework is in concordance with our vision for this book:

> The framework tracks learning and development through states and traits linked by life events and transitions that occur across successive years, from birth to death. The integration of … lifelong professional development … commences with the decision to pursue a career in medicine and ends with the decision to disengage from the field.

The framework examines definitions and constructs, checks its alignment with existing theories, and seeks to structure the often-unstructured trajectory of the years in practice. Thus, it facilitates planning, goal setting, and the enhancement of effective development that is also amenable to research and may be instrumental in quality improvement. Mazmanian et al. conclude:

> Recognizing long-term development and learning means acknowledging, tracking, and accounting for age-graded, history-graded and non-normative life events and transitions to improve our understandings of how physicians learn from developing and shaping their environment, while systematically comprising the ecology of human development, learning, and environment.

A similar message has recently been expressed by **Collins** and **Sanford**,[33] who also lament the lack of structure and attention to development beyond the formative years:

---

32 Mazmanian, P. E., Cervero, R. M., & Durning, S. J. (2021). Reimagining physician development and lifelong learning: An ecological framework. *Journal of Continuing Education in the Health Professions*, *41*(4), 291–298. https://doi.org/10.1097/CEH.0000000000000406

33 Collins, R. T., 2nd, & Sanford, R. (2021). The importance of formalized, lifelong physician career development: Making the case for a paradigm shift. *Academic Medicine: Journal of the Association of American Medical Colleges*, *96*(10), 1383–1388. https://doi.org/10.1097/ACM.0000000000004191

The lack of a philosophy of intentional, career-long individual development at academic medical centers reflects a narrow understanding of the implicit contract between employers and employees. The resulting gap leads the vast majority of physicians to fall short of their potential, further leading to long-term loss for the academic medical centers, their physicians, and society as a whole.

They propose:

A robust, iterative model for physician career development that goes beyond skills and knowledge maintenance toward leveraging a broad range of individual capabilities, needs, and contexts along the career lifespan. The model provides a means for harnessing physicians' strengths and passions in concert with the needs of their organization to create greater physician fulfillment and success.

The model described is an application of ADDIE (analyze, design, develop, implement, evaluate) to physician career development with subcomponents at each step. It is iterative and includes ongoing evaluation.

A survey of CME practices in the United States found that what physicians are looking for most in their choice of CME is up-to-date information or skills.[34] They feel comfortable identifying their CME needs and put professionalism as their last priority. Thus, the survey suggests, CME is usually about keeping current and less about finding a community of practice, and is not explicit about the inclusion of emotions, life stages, transitions, and identity.[35] A gap between theory and practice is evident here.[36] Several recent papers suggest fostering lifelong learning through more frequent assessment. We concur with the case made here

---

34 Cook, D. A., Blackman, M. J., Price, D. W., West, C. P., Borger, R. A., & Wittich, C. M. (2017). Professional development perceptions and practices among U.S. physicians: A cross-specialty national survey. *Academic Medicine: Journal of the Association of American Medical Colleges*, 92(9), 1335–1345. https://doi.org/10.1097/ACM.0000000000001624

35 Allen, L. M., Palermo, C., Armstrong, E., & Hay, M. (2019). Categorising the broad impacts of continuing professional development: A scoping review. *Medical Education*, 53(11), 1087–1099. https://doi.org/10.1111/medu.13922

36 Helmich, E., Yeh, H. M., Kalet, A., & Al-Eraky, M. (2017). Becoming a doctor in different cultures: Toward a cross-cultural approach to supporting professional identity formation in medicine. *Academic Medicine: Journal of the Association of American Medical Colleges*, 92(1), 58–62. https://doi.org/10.1097/ACM.0000000000001432

for revisiting CME so it shifts from "keeping updated" to maximizing one's potential. Some countries and systems have already taken steps in this direction, such as the United Kingdom's revalidation system.

Summary

The opening story describes the learning and teaching experience of a resident being coached by a senior clinician. It illustrates how, beyond knowledge and skills, the essence of a discipline may be transmitted on the job, and with a mutually transformative impact. This adult learning category delineates a career development stage model with a host of constructs, theories, and development-supporting pedagogies. It emphasizes the practice years and their developmental needs (whereas the first category and most of the literature address the formative years of medical school and residency). It also introduces learning as a social act, a socialization process—from clinical supervision and the classic dyadic mentoring of the opening story to communities of practice—whereby development is molded by the professional group and does not reside only as an intersubjective process (as in the first category). Furthermore, this category introduces lifelong learning and self-regulated learning, as well as burnout, resilience, narratives, the impact of technology (e.g., EMRs), a suggested midlife crisis, and the role of gender (further developed in Chapter 7). Finally, a recent ecological framework of this category, as well as a vision for structuring physician development during the practice years, are proposed. These recent voices state that practitioners in this phase of the professional life cycle often do not maximize their potential since their development is either ignored or almost taken for granted. In this category, more practical issues emerge. As CME lags, the understanding that it should aim at maximizing the practitioner's potential becomes apparent, and frameworks for structuring a change are offered.

REFERENCES

Allen, L. M., Palermo, C., Armstrong, E., & Hay, M. (2019). Categorising the broad impacts of continuing professional development: A scoping review. *Medical Education*, *53*(11), 1087–1099. https://doi.org/10.1111/medu.13922

Ballouk, R., Mansour, V., Dalziel, B., McDonald, J., & Hegazi, I. (2022). Medical students' self-regulation of learning in a blended learning environment: A systematic scoping review. *Medical Education Online*, *27*(1), 2029336. https://doi.org/10.1080/10872981.2022.2029336

Benner, P., Sutphen, M., Leonard-Kahn, V., & Day, L. (2008). Formation and everyday ethical comportment. *American Journal of Critical Care: An Official Publication, American Association of Critical-Care Nurses, 17*(5), 473–476.

Bennett, N. L., & Hotvedt, M. O. (1989). Stage of career. In R. D. Fox, P. E. Mazmanian, & R. W. Putnam (Eds.), *Changing and learning in the lives of physicians*. Praeger.

Bickel, J. (2016). Not too late to reinvigorate: How midcareer faculty can continue growing. *Academic Medicine: Journal of the Association of American Medical Colleges, 91*(12), 1601–1605. https://doi.org/10.1097/ACM.0000000000001310

Burton, J., & Launer, J. (Eds.). (2003). *Supervision and support in primary care*. CRC Press.

Cohen, R., Amiel, G. E., Tann, M., Shechter, A., Weingarten, M., & Reis, S. (2002). Performance assessment of community-based physicians: Evaluating the reliability and validity of a tool for determining CME needs. *Academic Medicine: Journal of the Association of American Medical Colleges, 77*(12 Pt 1), 1247–1254. https://doi.org/10.1097/00001888-200212000-00022

Collins, R. T., 2nd, & Sanford, R. (2021). The importance of formalized, lifelong physician career development: Making the case for a paradigm shift. *Academic Medicine: Journal of the Association of American Medical Colleges, 96*(10), 1383–1388. https://doi.org/10.1097/ACM.0000000000004191

Cook, D. A., Blachman, M. J., Price, D. W., West, C. P., Berger, R. A., & Wittich, C. M. (2017). Professional development perceptions and practices among U.S. physicians: A cross-specialty national survey. *Academic Medicine: Journal of the Association of American Medical Colleges, 92*(9), 1335–1345. https://doi.org/10.1097/ACM.0000000000001624

Dehning, S., Reiß, E., Krause, D., Gasperi, S., Meyer, S., Dargel, S., Müller, N., & Siebeck, M. (2014). Empathy in high-tech and high-touch medicine. *Patient Education and Counseling, 95*(2), 259–264. https://doi.org/10.1016/j.pec.2014.01.013

Foster, C. R., Dahill, L., Goleman, L. A., & Tolentino, B. W. (2005). *Educating clergy: Teaching practices and pastoral imagination*. Jossey-Bass.

Foster, K., & Roberts, C. (2016). The heroic and the villainous: A qualitative study characterising the role models that shaped senior doctors' professional identity. *BMC Medical Education, 16*(1), 206. https://doi.org/10.1186/s12909-016-0731-0

Fox, R. D. (2003). Continuing professional education. In J. W. Guthrie (Ed.), *Encyclopedia of education* (2nd ed.). Macmillan Reference.

Freeman, T. (2016). *McWhinney's textbook of family medicine* (4th ed.). Oxford University Press.

Hedlund, J., Forsythe, G. B., Horvath, J. A., Williams, W. M., Snook, S., & Sternberg, R. J. (2003). Identifying and assessing tacit knowledge: Understanding the practical intelligence of military leaders. *Leadership Quarterly, 14*(2), 117–140. https://doi.org/10.1016/S1048-9843(03)00006-7

Helmich, E., Yeh, H. M., Kalet, A., & Al-Eraky, M. (2017). Becoming a doctor in different cultures: Toward a cross-cultural approach to supporting professional identity formation in medicine. *Academic Medicine: Journal of the Association of American Medical Colleges, 92*(1), 58–62. https://doi.org/10.1097/ACM.0000000000001432

Jones, K., & Reis, S. (2010). Learning through vulnerability: A mentor-mentee experience. *Annals of Family Medicine, 8*(6), 552–555. https://doi.org/10.1370/afm.1165

Jones, W. A., Avant, R. F., Davis, N., Saultz, J., & Lyons, P. (2004). Task force report 3. Report of the task force on continuous personal, professional, and practice development in family medicine. *Annals of Family Medicine, 2*(Suppl 1), s65–s74. https://doi.org/10.1370/afm.136

Launer, J. (2007). Moving on from Balint: Embracing clinical supervision. *The British Journal of General Practice: The Journal of the Royal College of General Practitioners, 57*(536), 182–183.

Launer, J. (2019). Supervision, mentoring and coaching. In T. Swanwick, K. Forrest, & B. C. O'Brien (Eds.), *Understanding medical education—Evidence, theory, and practice*. John Wiley and Sons.

Lave, J., & Wenger, E. (1991). *Situated learning: Legitimate peripheral participation*. Cambridge University Press.

Le May, A. (2009). *Communities of practice in health and social care*. Wiley-Blackwell.

Little, M., & Midtling, J. E. (2011). *Becoming a family physician* (Softcover reprint of the original 1st ed. 1989). Springer.

Lockyer, J., de Groot, J., & Silver, I. (2016). Professional identity formation, the practicing physician and continuing professional development. In R. L. Cruess, S. R. Cruess, & Y. Steinert (Eds.), *Teaching medical professionalism: Supporting the development of a professional identity* (pp. 186–200). Cambridge University Press.

Löffler, C., Altiner, A., Blumenthal, S., Bruno, P., De Sutter, A., De Vos, B. J., Dinant, G. J., Duerden, M., Dunais, B., Egidi, G., Gibis, B., Melbye, H., Rouquier, F., Rosemann, T., Touboul-Lundgren, P., & Feldmeier, G. (2022). Challenges and opportunities for general practice specific CME in Europe—A narrative review of seven countries. *BMC Medical Education*, 22(1), 761. https://doi.org/10.1186/s12909-022-03832-7

Lovell, B. (2018). What do we know about coaching in medical education? A literature review. *Medical Education*, 52(4), 376–390. https://doi.org/10.1111/medu.13482

Mazmanian, P. E., Cervero, R. M., & Durning, S. J. (2021). Reimagining physician development and lifelong learning: An ecological framework. *Journal of Continuing Education in the Health Professions*, 41(4), 291–298. https://doi.org/10.1097/CEH.0000000000000406

Medalie, J. H. (1978). Introduction. In Medalie, J. H. (Ed.). *Family medicine: Principles and applications*. Williams & Wilkins.

Merriam, S. B., & Baumgartner, L. M. (2020). *Learning in adulthood: A comprehensive guide* (4th ed.). Jossey-Bass.

Neher, J. O., Gordon, K. C., Meyer, B., & Stevens, N. (1992). A five-step "microskills" model of clinical teaching. *Journal of the American Board of Family Practice*, 5(4), 419–424.

Palmer, P. J. (2017). *The courage to teach: Exploring the inner landscape of a teacher's life*. John Wiley & Sons.

Rabow, M. W., Remen, R. N., Parmelee, D. X., & Inui, T. S. (2010). Professional formation: Extending medicine's lineage of service into the next century. *Academic Medicine: Journal of the Association of American Medical Colleges*, 85(2), 310–317. https://doi.org/10.1097/ACM.0b013e3181c887f7

Ryan, A., Hickey, A., Harkin, D., Boland, F., Collins, M. E., & Doyle, F. (2023). Professional identity formation, professionalism, leadership and resilience (PILLAR) in medical students: Methodology and early results. *Journal of Medical Education and Curricular Development*, 10. https://doi.org/10.1177/23821205231198921

Super, D. E. (1957). *The psychology of careers*. Harper.

Sullivan, S. E. (1999). The changing nature of careers: A review and research agenda. *Journal of Management*, 25(3), 457–484. https://doi.org/10.1177/014920639902500308

Wenger, E. (1998). *Communities of practice: Learning, meaning, and identity*. Cambridge University Press. https://doi.org/10.1017/CBO9780511803932

CHAPTER 3

Expertise, clinical reasoning, deliberate practice, and phronesis

....

Such naches*

An evening (2007, Galilee, Israel)

I am a rural family doctor practicing in the Galilee, Israel. Some of my patients have known me for three decades and a few are close friends. I practice in a health center serving multiple small communities dispersed on the surrounding hilltops. Galit and Moshe, who live in Yad-Tal, a mile away from the practice, are dear friends and long-standing patients.

Recently, a routine appointment with Galit brought back memories of a profound story. Galit asked for a refill for Moshe's medications, I examined her back for her semiannual mole inspection and gave her a referral for orthotics. The printer clicked into action, I stamped the papers and prescriptions and handed them to her.

We were almost done when Galit said, "Hard times."

I knew she was referring to the shockingly rapid death, just a few days prior, of a neighbor of theirs. He had passed away while hospitalized in the same ward in which Gilad, Galit's elder son, had been years ago for his leukemia care.

She continued: "Gilad helped carry the coffin at the funeral. I looked at him, a tanned, healthy, strong young man – who has the guts to look death in the eye."

We stayed silent for a moment, then she got up to leave.

---

*   Naches—Joy: gratification, especially from children (Yiddish).

DOI: 10.1201/9781003507529-4

Early the next morning, I happened to receive an email from Michael, an old friend and family doctor living in Vancouver. Coincidentally, the content of his email happened to refer to events that involved Gilad, Galit, and Moshe, events that took place over seven years prior, halfway around the world.

On a busy morning in May 2000, Michael recalled, I called from Israel, a great sense of urgency in my voice as I told him about Gilad and his girlfriend Yam, who were touring Canada. I told him that Gilad had visited a walk-in clinic and been told that he had the flu and to go to bed.

I told Michael: "It does not sound like flu to me! Would you be able to see him please?"

Michael changed his schedule and saw Gilad and Yam shortly after the phone call. As Michael told it: Gilad was approaching down the hall, and it was obvious that he was a very sick young man. He was pale, sweating, and walking with great effort. He had a high fever and elevated and weak pulse. His lymph nodes were enlarged and his spleen as well. In fact, for a man as sick as he was, it seemed strange that he could even walk.

Michael sent him to a nearby lab and was called shortly thereafter with the news he feared. The white cell count was 186,000—and those white cells were very immature. Gilad had acute myelogenous leukemia, an extremely dangerous form of leukemia.

Michael could not remember the exact details of how quickly he had gotten Gilad to Vancouver Hospital and onto the leukemia ward, only that it happened fast.

Apart from Gilad's precarious state, the other striking feature for Michael was the relationship between Gilad and Yam. Yam was loving and efficient and focused. It was she who got Gilad to do what was necessary, as he was much too sick to make judgments on his own.

Later that day, Michael visited the ward and found Gilad and Yam in isolation in a special room for patients whose defenses are so weak that they need to be protected from infection. Going in and out was closely controlled. The ward nurses coming in and out of the room with an efficient, no-nonsense demeanor were warm and compassionate in spite of their protective gear.

I did not need Michael's email and recollections to be transported back to these heart-wrenching days. I have known Gilad and the family forever; we have shared multiple mundane moments and extraordinary feats. For example, for years Galit and Moshe struggled with infertility and decided to adopt Gilad, only to go on to have two biological children. As friends, they supported me through a painful divorce and rejoiced in the blossoming of my second marriage.

Breaking the news of Gilad's leukemia to Galit and Moshe was terrible. I recall driving the short distance from my home to theirs and saying those ominous words, "I am sorry to have to tell you that Gilad is very, very sick." It was almost as if my own child was severely afflicted. Distance amplified the concern and apprehension. It was one of the most difficult moments in my life, too. I kept in close telephone and email touch with Michael and the physician head of the leuke-mia service. A remarkable, transnational, and collaborative planning for Gilad's treatment took place, with leukemia specialists from my local tertiary service at Rambam Medical Center in Haifa involved. Gilad's treatment began urgently. He received blood and platelet transfusions, and as soon as his severe anemia and platelet absence were in check, his treatment with chemotherapy for the leukemia began.

Unfortunately, Gilad's response to the chemotherapy was cataclysmic. The drug killed Gilad's white cells in such great numbers and so quickly that his body could not handle the breakdown products of the destroyed white cells. Gilad went into respiratory and kidney failure. In short order he was on a respirator and on renal dialysis. Had he not been in such great shape, so well supported by Yam, and under superb care, he would have died. …

This deterioration and need for intensive care prompted mortal fear on our side of the globe. I recall imploring Michael to multiply his efforts (a reflection of my helplessness and fear, no doubt) to save Gilad. It may sound unreal, yet thanks to the wonders of information technology—the constant communication via phone and email with Michael and those attending Gilad at the hospital, looking up the hospital's website and finding a floor plan, and finally a dose of creative imagina-tion rendered feverish by the strong emotions—I felt virtually present in that room and ward with Gilad on a ventilator, Yam at his bedside, and Michael and those remarkable nurses and physicians busy saving his life.

Yam "lived" in the isolation room for the month of Gilad's stay in Vancouver. Soon Gilad's parents, first Galit and later Moshe, arrived. Michael wrote: "It was our pleasure to know them, sensible and strong parents, who obviously loved Yam. Galit, as I remember it, arrived at the worst phase of the illness, with life in the balance. Yet she was calm and immediately helpful and supportive of Yam. I felt that I got to know Yam, Moshe, and Galit well. Gilad was rather quiet and taciturn. I think he was putting all his energy into getting better. But though he did not talk much to me, he clearly was in love with Yam and glowed in her presence."

Michael is an old friend, yet we could not even in our wildest dreams have imagined our relationship becoming handy in such circumstances. I have found a note that I wrote to Michael some time ago: "We have not met often, nor for prolonged periods. In the last years we have had mostly a virtual relationship. But oh, can this virtual bond be real! Take this example: I was called by a friend-patient one morning telling me that her son was sick in Vancouver. You became his family doctor, hosted his parents who flew in, kept in constant communication with me, and returned him safely home (Gilad received an autologous bone marrow trans-plantation and went into full remission for more than six years). I felt, thanks to you, the rest of the medical team, and the wonders of information technology as if I was there. (We should write this up one day.)"

Here we are writing it up.

Subsequently, this drama of terror and healing reached its climax with Gilad and Yam getting married on a glorious spring night in 2004. They have had two [now four] lovely children since. Michael wrote: "When my wife Bonnie and I were invited to the wedding we were so pleased and proud to have had a little to do with this lovely couple – and we are still kicking ourselves for not being able to go to the wedding. And now the baby!! And the photos from the proud grandparents. Such *naches*!" Indeed, such joy!

In the busy life of practitioner-academics such as Michael and myself, we encounter our share of death, suffering, and futility. Celebrating this miracle of friendship, love, and healing is re-moralizing, for us and, we hope, for all.[1]

* * *

The opening story of this category displays how lifesaving expertise is mobilized across oceans. Shmuel Reis, co-author of this book, tells Michael Klein, a Vancouver-based family medicine professor and a friend, "It does not sound like flu to me," based on his phone conversation with Gilad's mother. Such pattern recognition and handling of the emergency are hallmarks of expertise and phronesis.

STAGES OF MEDICAL EXPERTISE DEVELOPMENT AND THE ZONE OF PROXIMAL DEVELOPMENT

While a definition for expertise in medicine remains controversial, the notion of expertise as an ultimate possible developmental stage in any domain is well established.[2,3,4] "According to expertise theories, pattern matching and effortlessly retrieved memories of previously executed actions eventually, naturally replace knowledge and consideration of

1   Reis, S., & Klein, M. (2011). Such naches. *Patient Education and Counseling, 83*(1), 45–46. https://doi.org/10.1016/j.pec.2010.03.012. Reproduced with permission from Elsevier.

2   Carraccio, C. L., Benson, B. J., Nixon, L. J., & Derstine, P. L. (2008). From the educational bench to the clinical bedside: Translating the Dreyfus developmental model to the learning of clinical skills. *Academic Medicine: Journal of the Association of American Medical Colleges, 83*(8), 761–767. https://doi.org/10.1097/ACM.0b013e31817eb632

3   Krackov, S. K., & Pohl, H. (2011). Building expertise using the deliberate practice curriculum-planning model. *Medical Teacher, 33*(7), 570–575. https://doi.org/10.3109/0142159X.2011.578172

4   Dreyfus, H., & Dreyfus, S. E. (1987). *Mind over machine: The power of human intuition and expertise in the era of the computer.* Free Press.

rules,"[5] is one description. Nevertheless, this domain continues to be extensively researched and popularized (by, among others, the maxim designating 10,000 hours needed for expertise development).[6] It is generally accepted that achieving expertise in any given field requires extensive, sustained, and **deliberate practice** of its necessary skills.[7,8,9] An expertise developmental model for medicine is associated with **Hubert Dreyfus** and **Stuart Dreyfus**, who describe the following stages: **novice, advanced beginner, competent, proficient, expert, and master** (Figure 3.1).

Dunphy and **Williamson**[10] supply a detailed description of medicine's "pursuit of expertise." Experts recognize complex patterns, possess additional cognitive space available for deliberation, use metacognitive mentoring, and have high levels of contextual flexibility. They also quote **Vygotsky**'s notion of the **zone of proximal development** (ZPD) as the "crucible" of professional growth. ZPD is where a disorienting dilemma arises: vulnerability and sometimes helplessness may prevail, and discomfort and liminality are experienced. Yet, the ZPD is where change and transformation occur. Is this where learning to heal in Weston terms takes place? Is this zone analogous to the liminal space (Chapter 1)? We expand on the ZPD further in this chapter and in Chapter 10.

The most extensively researched domain of medical expertise is the development of clinical reasoning.[11,12] Other frequently researched

5   Ericsson, K. A. (2015). Acquisition and maintenance of medical expertise: A perspective from the expert-performance approach with deliberate practice. *Academic Medicine: Journal of the Association of American Medical Colleges*, 90(11), 1471–1486. https://doi.org/10.1097/ACM.0000000000000939

6   Gladwell, M. (2008). *Outliers: The story of success.* Little, Brown and Company.

7   Dreyfus, H. (2006, September 9). *From novice to world discloser.* Paper presented at the Accreditation Council for Graduate Medical Education Design Conference on the Learning Environment, Chicago, IL.

8   Schei, E., Knoop, H. S., Gismervik, M. N., Mylopoulos, M., & Boudreau, J. D. (2019). Stretching the comfort zone: Using early clinical contact to influence professional identity formation in medical students. *Journal of Medical Education and Curricular Development*, 6. https://doi.org/10.1177/2382120519843875

9   Groot, F., Jonker, G., Rinia, M., Ten Cate, O., & Hoff, R. G. (2020). Simulation at the frontier of the zone of proximal development: A test in acute care for inexperienced learners. *Academic Medicine: Journal of the Association of American Medical Colleges*, 95(7), 1098–1105. https://doi.org/10.1097/ACM.0000000000003265

10 Dunphy, B. C., & Williamson, S. L. (2004). In pursuit of expertise: Toward an educational model for expertise development. *Advances in Health Sciences Education: Theory and Practice*, 9(2), 107–127. https://doi.org/10.1023/B:AHSE.0000027436.17220.9c

11 Groopman, J. (2007). *How doctors think.* Houghton Mifflin.

12 Montgomery, K. (2005). *How doctors think: Clinical judgment and the practice of medicine.* Oxford University Press.

List 1

Principles of the Dreyfus and Dreyfus Model of Skill Development Applied to the Development of a Physician's Competence

Novice
- Is rule driven
- Uses analytic reasoning and rules to link cause and effect
- Has little ability to filter or prioritize information, so synthesis is difficult at best and the big picture is elusive

Advanced beginner
- Is able to sort through rules and information to decide what is relevant on the basis of past experience
- Uses both analytic reasoning and pattern recognition to solve problems
- Is able to abstract from concrete and specific information to more general aspects of a problem

Competent
- Emotional buy-in allows the learner to feel an appropriate level of responsibility
- More expansive experience tips the balance in clinical reasoning from methodical and analytic to more readily identifiable pattern recognition of common clinical problem presentations
- Sees the big picture
- Complex or uncommon problems still require reliance on analytic reasoning

Proficient
- Breadth of past experience allows one to rely on pattern recognition of illness presentation such that clinical problem-solving seems intuitive
- Still needs to fall back to methodical and analytic reasoning for managing problems because exhaustive number of permutations and responses to management have provided less experience in this regard than in illness recognition
- Is comfortable with evolving situations; able to extrapolate from a known situation to an unknown situation (capable)
- Can live with ambiguity

Expert
- Thought, feeling, and action align into intuitive problem recognition and intuitive situational responses and management
- Is open to notice the unexpected
- Is clever
- Is perceptive in discriminating features that do not fit a recognizable pattern

Master
- Exercises practical wisdom
- Goes beyond the big picture and sees a bigger picture of the culture and context of each situation
- Has a deep level of commitment to the work
- Has great concern for right and wrong decisions; this fosters emotional engagement
- Is intensely motivated by emotional engagement to pursue ongoing learning and improvement
- Reflects in, on, and for action

FIGURE 3.1 Dreyfus and Dreyfus Model of Expertise (Reproduced with permission. Carraccio, C. L., Benson, B. J., Nixon, L. J., & Derstine, P. L. (2008). From the educational bench to the clinical bedside: Translating the Dreyfus developmental model to the learning of clinical skills. *Academic Medicine: Journal of the Association of American Medical Colleges, 83*(8), 761–767. https://doi.org/10.1097/ACM.0b013e31817eb632.)

domains include surgical skills[13] and visual interpretation skills (radiology).[14]

Dall'Alba, an aforementioned critic of the stage model (see Chapter 1), postulates that it is understanding, through practice, that begets "professional ways of being," which integrate knowing, acting, and being. Further, she emphasizes the view that **many professionals do not achieve the expert stage**, explaining this **by absence of enough critical reflection and deliberate practice** to support the development of expert or master embodied understanding.

For nearly two decades, the expertise construct, or rather the notion of exceptional performance, has been tied to the research of **Anders Ericsson**.[15] In a series of papers and a book titled *Peak*,[16] he proposes that behind expertise is prolonged deliberate practice (DP). He redefines the criteria for genuine DP and introduces the 10,000-hour rule, later popularized by **Gladwell**. He and others describe three stages of expertise development:[17,18] the first, through usual modes of teaching and learning, such as lectures, books, conferences, and so on; the second, aimed at mastery, in which exposure and repetitive practice are employed to gain automaticity of skill application and to reach a minimum performance threshold; and third, **deliberate practice** within **an expert performance**

13 Dearani, J. A., Gold, M., Leibovich, B. C., Ericsson, K. A., Khabbaz, K. R., Foley, T. A., Julsrud, P. R., Matsumoto, J. M., & Daly, R. C. (2017). The role of imaging, deliberate practice, structure, and improvisation in approaching surgical perfection. *Journal of Thoracic and Cardiovascular Surgery, 154*(4), 1329–1336. https://doi.org/10.1016/j.jtcvs.2017.04.045

14 Waite, S., Farooq, Z., Grigorian, A., Sistrom, C., Kolla, S., Mancuso, A., Martinez-Conde, S., Alexander, R. G., Kantor, A., & Macknik, S. L. (2020). A review of perceptual expertise in radiology—How it develops, how we can test it, and why humans still matter in the era of artificial intelligence. *Academic Radiology, 27*(1), 26–38. https://doi.org/10.1016/j.acra.2019.08.018

15 Ericsson, K. A. (2015). Acquisition and maintenance of medical expertise: A perspective from the expert-performance approach with deliberate practice. *Academic Medicine: Journal of the Association of American Medical Colleges, 90*(11), 1471–1486. https://doi.org/10.1097/ACM.0000000000000939

16 Ericsson, K. A., & Pool, R. (2016). *Peak: How all of us can achieve extraordinary things*. Vintage.

17 Ericsson, K. A., Nandagopal, K., & Roring, R. W. (2009). Toward a science of exceptional achievement: Attaining superior performance through deliberate practice. *Annals of the New York Academy of Sciences, 1172*, 199–217. https://doi.org/10.1196/annals.1393.001

18 Ericsson, K. A., & Harwell, K. W. (2019). Deliberate practice and proposed limits on the effects of practice on the acquisition of expert performance: Why the original definition matters and recommendations for future research. *Frontiers in Psychology, 10*, 2396. https://doi.org/10.3389/fpsyg.2019.02396

approach, aiming for the highest possible functioning.[19] The latter is not satisfied by routine expertise (the automatic, fluid performance in routine situations). Rather, this third stage seeks **adaptive expertise,** the ability to achieve peak performance in novel and challenging situations.[20]

Ericsson postulated that adaptive expertise is based on mental representations (Figure 3.2) that are formed and refined through deliberate practice. These representations span what should be done (before), what is done (during), and what should happen after (the desired performance). These empirical and theoretical premises are supported by fMRI (functional magnetic resonance imaging) and electrophysiological

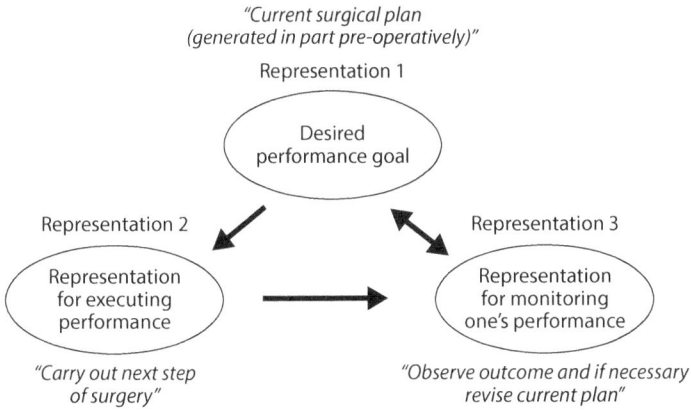

"Current surgical plan (generated in part pre-operatively)"

Representation 1

Desired performance goal

Representation 2

Representation 3

Representation for executing performance

Representation for monitoring one's performance

"Carry out next step of surgery"

"Observe outcome and if necessary revise current plan"

FIGURE 3.2 Three Types of Internal Representations That Mediate Expert Performance and Its Continued Improvement during Practice (Reproduced with permission from Wolters Kluwer Health, Inc. Ericsson, K. A. 2015. Acquisition and maintenance of medical expertise: A perspective from the expert-performance approach with deliberate practice. *Academic Medicine: Journal of the Association of American Medical Colleges,* 90(11), 1471–1486. https://doi.org/10.1097/ACM.0000000000000939.)

---

19 Ericsson, K. A., Hoffman, R. R., Kozbelt, A., & Williams, A. M. (Eds.). (2018). *The Cambridge handbook of expertise and expert performance* (2nd ed.). Cambridge University Press. https://doi.org/10.1017/9781316480748

20 Betinol, E., Murphy, S., & Regehr, G. (2023). Exploring the development of adaptive expertise through the lens of threshold concepts. *Medical Education,* 57(2), 142–150. https://doi.org/10.1111/medu.14887

measurements that lend further support to these constructs.[21,22] In addition, pedagogies to accelerate expertise development have been described and show positive results.[23,24] Different disciplines, such as surgery, imaging, and anesthesia, use these approaches to take a fresh look at their expertise development programs and modify them based on the DP framework.[25,26] This fresh look identifies that **most specialist physicians (by formal degree) do not reach the level of master or adaptive expert,** since they are not engaging in DP. The notion of the ZPD is again associated with developmental transitions, as well as with any challenging new learning. Finally, simulation has catapulted training for expertise to new levels of sophistication, especially in the surgical domain as it perfectly supports deliberate practice.[27] Moreover, options for artificial intelligence and 3D printing add additional preparatory phases of elaborate mental representations before performing complex operations.

An additional elaboration on the transition from routine to adaptive expertise is the introduction of the **master adaptive learner (MAL)**

21 Li, Q., Wang, X., Wang, S., Xie, Y., Li, X., Xie, Y., & Li, S. (2019). Dynamic reconfiguration of the functional brain network after musical training in young adults. *Brain Structure & Function*, *224*(5), 1781–1795. https://doi.org/10.1007/s00429-019-01867-z

22 Durning, S. J., Costanzo, M. E., Beckman, T. J., Artino, A. R., Jr, Roy, M. J., van der Vleuten, C., Holmboe, E. S., Lipner, R. S., & Schuwirth, L. (2016). Functional neuroimaging correlates of thinking flexibility and knowledge structure in memory: Exploring the relationships between clinical reasoning and diagnostic thinking. *Medical Teacher*, *38*(6), 570–577. https://doi.org/10.3109/0142159X.2015.1047755

23 Causer, J., Barach, P., & Williams, A. M. (2014). Expertise in medicine: Using the expert performance approach to improve simulation training. *Medical Education*, *48*(2), 115–123. https://doi.org/10.1111/medu.12306

24 Rissmiller, B., Castro, D., Minard, C. G., Sur, M., Roy, K., Turner, T., & Thammasithoon, S. (2019). The diagnostic expertise acceleration module (DEAM): Promoting the formation of organized knowledge. *Medical Education Online*, *24*(1). https://doi.org/10.1080/10872981.2019.1679945

25 Schmidt, P. C., & Fenner, D. E. (2020). Deliberate practice: Applying the expert performance approach to gynecologic surgical training. *Clinical Obstetrics and Gynecology*, *63*(2), 295–304. https://doi.org/10.1097/GRF.0000000000000509

26 Hastings, R. H., & Rickard, T. C. (2015). Deliberate practice for achieving and maintaining expertise in anesthesiology. *Anesthesia and Analgesia*, *120*(2), 449–459. https://doi.org/10.1213/ANE.0000000000000526

27 McGaghie, W. C., Issenberg, S. B., Cohen, E. R., Barsuk, J. H., & Wayne, D. B. (2011). Does simulation-based medical education with deliberate practice yield better results than traditional clinical education? A meta-analytic comparative review of the evidence. *Academic Medicine: Journal of the Association of American Medical Colleges*, *86*(6), 706–711. https://doi.org/10.1097/ACM.0b013e318217e119

concept.[28] This construct integrates lifelong learning skills into four stages: planning, learning, assessing, and adjusting. Crucial cognitive skills are critical thinking and reflection, which support the necessary metacognition: "Combining critical thinking and reflection allows a learner to be intentional about their own learning and to understand whether the learning is effective."

CLINICAL REASONING

Two books published in the early 2000s with identical titles address their eponymous topic: *How Doctors Think*. The first, more scholarly, was written by **Montgomery** (2005). The second, written by **Groopman** (2007), enjoyed bestseller status. Both of these books, and the literature on physician expertise as a whole, address clinical reasoning, described as an integration of analytic and pattern-based recognition processes.[29,30] Here, too, a four-stage developmental process is described by **Schmidt** et al. whereby causal networks are initially organized and synthesized through the formative years until illness scripts emerge, stored so that they can be instantiated when the clinician encounters the next clinical challenge.[31] Both the Dreyfus levels of mastery and mature clinical reasoning are characterized by **phronesis**, an Aristotelian term describing hard-earned practical wisdom. This wisdom enables the professional to apply decision-making and interventions masterfully to particular problems and persons, such as when the best approach for the same biomedical situation may be diametrically opposed depending on context.

Groopman asks questions such as: Do different doctors think differently? Why do even experienced doctors make mistakes? Is there one "best" way to think? He supplies some answers: "Expertise is largely

28 Cutrer, W. B., Miller, B., Pusic, M. V., Mejicano, G., Mangrulkar, R. S., Gruppen, L. D., Hawkins, R. E., Skochelak, S. E., & Moore, D. E., Jr. (2017). Fostering the development of master adaptive learners: A conceptual model to guide skill acquisition in medical education. *Academic Medicine: Journal of the Association of American Medical Colleges*, 92(1), 70–75. https://doi.org/10.1097/ACM.0000000000001323

29 Schmidt, H. G., Norman, G. R., & Boshuizen, H. P. (1990). A cognitive perspective on medical expertise: Theory and implication. *Academic Medicine: Journal of the Association of American Medical Colleges*, 65(10), 611–621. https://doi.org/10.1097/00001888-199010000-00001

30 Mamede, S., & Schmidt, H. G. (2004). The structure of reflective practice in medicine. *Medical Education*, 38(12), 1302–1308. https://doi.org/10.1111/j.1365-2929.2004.01917.x

31 Schmidt, P. C., & Fenner, D. E. (2020). Deliberate practice: Applying the expert performance approach to gynecologic surgical training. *Clinical Obstetrics and Gynecology*, 63(2), 295–304. https://doi.org/10.1097/GRF.0000000000000509

acquired not only by sustained practice but by receiving feedback that helps you understand your technical errors and misguided decisions." Experts use **heuristics** (mental shortcuts) and develop hypotheses from very incomplete data, as Groopman quotes **Schön**:

> Because of some puzzling, troubling, interesting phenomena, a physician expresses uncertainty, takes the time to reflect, and allows himself to be vulnerable. Then he restructures the problem. This is the key to the art of dealing with situations of uncertainty, instability, uniqueness, and value conflict.

This characterization also rings true for a learning and development opportunity such as the ZPD. The components of disorienting dilemmas are often multidimensional, with conflicting values and contradictory truths. Their inherent uncertainty challenges the comfort zone, engendering vulnerability, sometimes helplessness. The ZPD is where, through reflection, mentoring, and sharing with a community of practice, developmental breakthroughs may emerge. However, these transitional points may also be where disability and developmental arrest or decline take place.

Montgomery identifies **clinical judgment** as the core of medical expertise. What characterizes the care of patients is phronesis. She stresses that medicine is scientific but not a science. While scientific and technological advances continuously refine clinical problems and provide solutions, they reduce but do not eliminate uncertainty, so that physicians still work in situations of inescapable uncertainty. This uncertainty is "ritualized, professionalized, and then for the most part ignored." Montgomery postulates that the first two years of a typical North American medical school (circa 1980s to 2005) were "crammed to overflowing with what is known," while clerkship, traditionally the latter two years, prepared learners to act in uncertain situations. Medical education transforms students of science into **reliable and practical reasoners**. Novices "must learn not only what course of action will be most likely to benefit the patient (even when choices are not good ones) but also what to do when information is conflicting or unavailable." This duality thus renders medical education a moral as well as intellectual enterprise.

Medical education is also experiential, behavioral, and in important ways covert. The misunderstanding of the epistemology of medicine has led to a harsh, often brutal education, unnecessarily impersonal clinical practice, dissatisfied patients, and disheartened physicians. Montgomery, who pioneered attention to the pervasive presence of narrative in clinical practice (see Chapter 5), readily observed the case-based narrative method by which clinicians organize and transmit knowledge. Clinical knowing "is particular, experiential, and conventionally agreed upon ...

physicians … rely on skill and judgment that are taught and practiced, improved and clarified case by case. … [It is] detail-driven wisdom."

In their research on clinical reasoning and diagnostic accuracy, **Mamede** et al. repeatedly show that these depend on deliberate reflection. Better reflectors are better diagnosticians. This aspect is expanded upon in Chapter 5.[32,33]

METACOGNITION, INTUITION, PHRONESIS, AND TRANSFORMATIVE EXPERTISE

In 2006, medical educator **Mark Quirk**[34] wrote a book on expertise development, postulating that mastery is about the development of **metacognition and intuition**. Quirk, in concordance with Montgomery[35] and Groopman[36], asserts the medical expert's need to instantiate diagnosis, treatment, and action plans in real time, with time and resource constraints. He believes that this is achieved through the cultivation and ongoing refinement and development of metacognition and intuition. **Carraccio** et al.,[37] quoting the Dreyfus novice to master model and referencing the clinical reasoning development stages of Schmidt et al., translate the Dreyfus model to the learning of clinical skills, which are refined and evolve throughout the stages of the physician's life cycle.

Although clinical reasoning and skills are the central focus of the literature reviewed up to this point, more reflective aspects of physician expertise do appear, such as in the work of Dall'Alba, Groopman,

32 Mamede, S., Hautz, W. E., Berendonk, C., Hautz, S. C., Sauter, T. C., Rotgans, J., Zwaan, L., & Schmidt, H. G. (2020). Think twice: Effects on diagnostic accuracy of returning to the case to reflect upon the initial diagnosis. *Academic Medicine: Journal of the Association of American Medical Colleges, 95*(8), 1223–1229. https://doi.org/10.1097/ACM.0000000000003153

33 Mamede, S., Figueiredo-Soares, T., Elói Santos, S. M., de Faria, R. M. D., Schmidt, H. G., & van Gog, T. (2019). Fostering novice students' diagnostic ability: The value of guiding deliberate reflection. *Medical Education, 53*(6), 628–637. https://doi.org/10.1111/medu.13829

34 Quirk, M. (2006). *Intuition and metacognition in medical education: Keys to developing expertise.* Springer.

35 Montgomery, K. (2005). *How doctors think: Clinical judgment and the practice of medicine.* Oxford University Press.

36 Groopman, J. (2007). *How doctors think.* Houghton Mifflin.

37 Carraccio, C. L., Benson, B. J., Nixon, L. J., & Derstine, P. L. (2008). From the educational bench to the clinical bedside: Translating the Dreyfus developmental model to the learning of clinical skills. *Academic Medicine: Journal of the Association of American Medical Colleges, 83*(8), 761–767. https://doi.org/10.1097/ACM.0b013e31817eb632

and Quirk. Aristotle considered phronesis to be one of the intellectual virtues or excellences of mind. He distinguished it from the two other virtues of episteme and techne (scientific knowledge and technical knowledge, respectively, in today's terms). Phronesis is associated with ethics. It juggles values and practical judgment and is informed by reflection.[38]

Engeström's cultural–historical activity theory (CHAT) is a framework for examining transformations in education, work, and communities, with multiple applications and interventions in healthcare. In his 2018 book, he introduces a transition from individual to collective expertise and delineates **the zone of proximal development of medical expertise,** proposing three spearheads that should beget **collaborative and transformative expertise:** knotworking, object and activity work systems, and expansive learning. This view expands the view of expertise

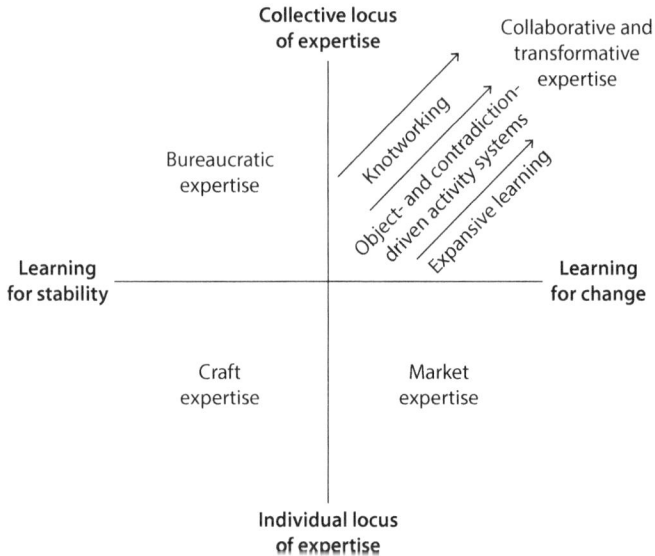

FIGURE 3.3 The Zone of Proximal Development of Expertise (Reproduced with permission from Cambridge University Press. Engeström, Y. 2018. *Expertise in transition: Expansive learning in medical work.* Cambridge University Press. https://doi.org/10.1017/9781139023009.)

toward a collective expertise and a focus on change (Figure 3.3). In other words, scholarly work that synergizes different constructs of our identified categories is available, validating our analysis and facilitating the development of integrated frameworks with both theoretical and practical ramifications.[39,40]

In this vein, **Paes** et al. conducted qualitative research to elucidate the developmental stages of phronesis when solving complex medical problems.[41,42] They found that self-efficacy and self-regulated learning are the key internal factors driving this development and suggest a three-stage model that can serve as a basis for educational and system interventions to foster phronesis (Figure 3.4).

In *Phronesis as Professional Knowledge*, **Kinsella** and **Pitman** define phronesis as "practical wisdom or knowledge of the proper ends of life."[43] **Frank**'s chapter in their book, titled "Reflective Healthcare Practice,"[44] begins with the question, "Who is sick?" indicating that medicine reduces the answer to this question to whoever has a diagnosable illness. This reduction stops us from thinking where wisdom needs to emerge and overcome knowledge. Frank postulates that a health professional has a choice between seeing her workday as one long checklist, thereby refraining from looking back or around to successfully complete her daily work, or engaging in sufficient reflection so that, along the way, phronesis—which Frank emphasizes as the assuming of personal responsibility based on experience—may develop.

39 Shachak, A., Buchanan, F., & Kuziemsky, C. (2024). When rules turn into tools: An activity theory-based perspective on implementation processes and unintended consequences. *Healthcare Management Forum*, 37(3), 177–182. https://doi.org/10.1177/08404704241233169

40 Shah, A. P., Walker, K. A., Hawick, L., Walker, K. G., & Cleland, J. (2023). Scratching beneath the surface: How organisational culture influences curricular reform. *Medical Education*, 57(7), 668–678. https://doi.org/10.1111/medu.14994

41 Paes, P. (2019). Practical wisdom, a dormant character in medical education? *Medical Education*, 53(5), 428–429. https://doi.org/10.1111/medu.13832

42 Paes, P., Leat, D., & Stewart, J. (2019). Complex decision making in medical training: Key internal and external influences in developing practical wisdom. *Medical Education*, 53(2), 165–174. https://doi.org/10.1111/medu.13767

43 Kinsella, E. A., & Pitman, A. (Eds.). (2012). *Phronesis as professional knowledge: Practical wisdom in the professions.* Sense Publishers. https://doi.org/10.1007/978-94-6091-731-8

44 Frank, A. W. (2012). Reflective healthcare practice: Claims, phronesis and dialogue. In E. A. Kinsella & A. Pitman (Eds.), *Phronesis as professional knowledge: Practical wisdom in the professions* (pp. 53–60). Sense Publishers. https://doi.org/10.1007/978-94-6091-731-8

THE DEVELOPMENT OF PRACTICAL WISDOM - A CONCEPTUAL MODEL

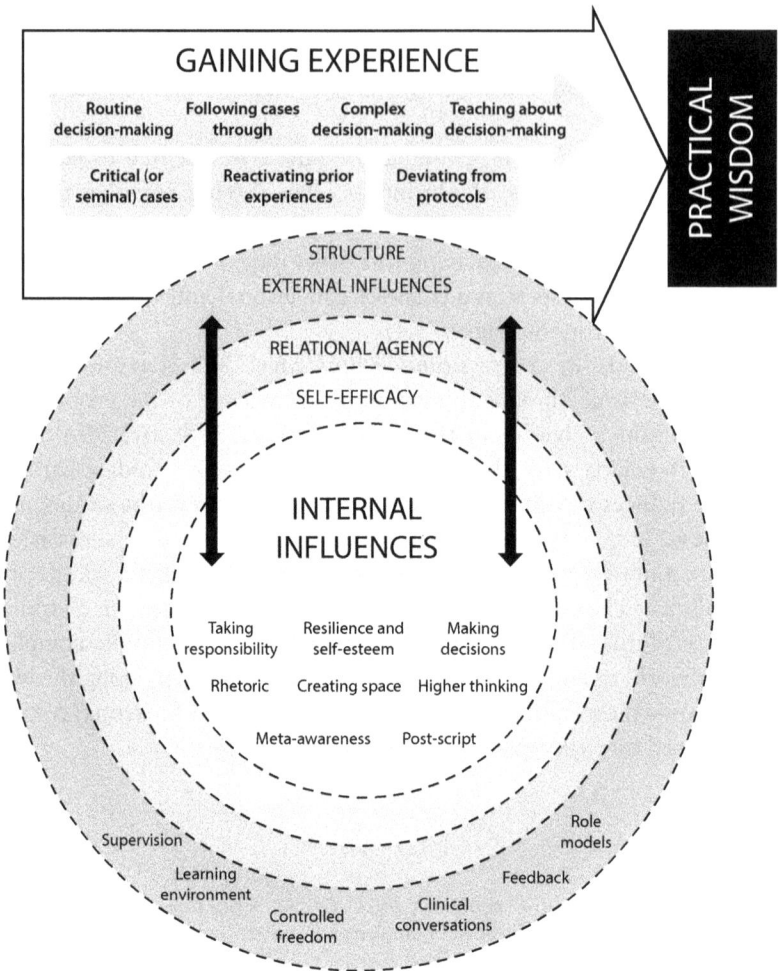

GAINING EXPERIENCE

| Routine decision-making | Following cases through | Complex decision-making | Teaching about decision-making |

| Critical (or seminal) cases | Reactivating prior experiences | Deviating from protocols |

PRACTICAL WISDOM

STRUCTURE
EXTERNAL INFLUENCES

RELATIONAL AGENCY

SELF-EFFICACY

INTERNAL INFLUENCES

| Taking responsibility | Resilience and self-esteem | Making decisions |

| Rhetoric | Creating space | Higher thinking |

| Meta-awareness | Post-script |

Supervision

Role models

Learning environment

Feedback

Controlled freedom

Clinical conversations

FIGURE 3.4 Complex Decision Making in Medical Training—Influences in Developing Practical Wisdom (Reproduced with permission from Wolters Kluwer Health, Inc. and the Copyright Clearance Center. Paes, P., Leat, D., & Stewart, J. 2019. Complex decision making in medical training: Key internal and external influences in developing practical wisdom. *Medical Education*, 53(2), 165–174. https://doi.org/10.1111/medu.13767.)

To Frank, reflection often begins with a pause. He enumerates six requirements from the professional during this time. First, **the practical,** is an outcome of the clinical encounter. Second, **the professional,** standing up to colleagues, and institutional and personal expectations. Third,

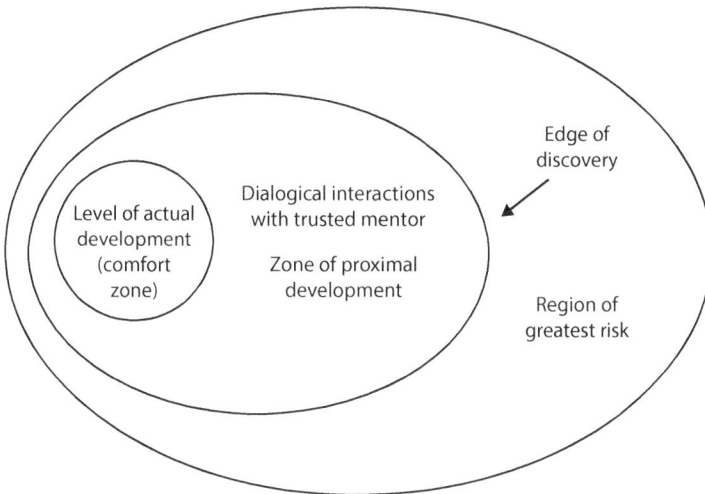

FIGURE 3.5 Learning Zones, Dialogue, and Risk, Modeled after Work by Vygotsky (Reproduced with permission. Kumagai, A. K. 2022. Discomfort, doubt, and the edge of learning. *Academic Medicine: Journal of the Association of American Medical Colleges*, 97(5), 649–654. https:// doi.org/10.1097/ACM.0000000000004588.)

the scientific, is operating according to evidence that supports the professional's actions. Fourth, **the commercial,** is fulfilling the expectation of her employer. Fifth, **the ethical,** what one should not do, in the bioethical sense. Finally, sixth, **the moral** is the expectation for a moral act such as bearing witness to the patient's suffering. The latter is sometimes framed in **Petty**'s words: "Don't just do something—stand there!"[45] It also reminds of Kleinman's statement that practitioners see themselves as "students of human nature, teachers of moral wisdom" (as discussed in the Introduction).

APORIA AND THE ZONE OF PROXIMAL DEVELOPMENT

Kumagai addresses the ZPD as an issue of "discomfort, doubt and the edge of learning" (Figure 3.5). A learner's level of actual development is their emotional and psychological security, mediated by personal identity, background, and experience. When physicians encounter human suffering, struggle, and pain to a degree they may have never experienced, they are forced out of their comfort zone and into a state of

---

45 Petty, T. L. (1979). Don't just do something—stand there! *Archives of Internal Medicine*, 139(8), 920–921. https://doi.org/10.1001/archinte.1979.03630450062020

	Objectives	Outcome
Informative	Information, skills	Experts
Formative	Socialisation, values	Professionals
Transformative	Leadership attributes	Change agents

FIGURE 3.6 Levels of Learning

aporia, of impasse and puzzlement, for which they may be completely unprepared. *Exposure to traumatic events or situations without mediated support or supervision may place learners in the region of greatest psychological risk.* However, with the help of a trusted mentor, their ZPD may be extended and enriched, and their **edge of discovery** may be pushed far beyond their preconceived expectations.

In addition to the aforementioned literature, the growing visibility of reflection as foundational for physician development and practice is also evident through growing availability of guidance on its application.[46]

THE INFORMATIVE–FORMATIVE–TRANSFORMATIVE PARADIGM

This chapter would be incomplete without touching on the informative–formative–transformative paradigm, also attributed to Kegan.[47] This framework was adopted by the *Lancet* Commission on Medical Education as best fit for the goal of health professional formation. The informative level is where professional knowledge and skills are acquired, producing experts. The formative level is where professional identity is formed and begets professionals. And, the transformative level is where attention to context and leadership is gained, resulting in "enlightened change agents" (Figure 3.6).

46 Sandars, J., Allan, D., & Price, J. (2023). Reflective practice by health professions educators to enhance learning and teaching: AMEE Guide No. 166. *Medical Teacher*, 1–10. https://doi.org/10.1080/0142159X.2023.2259071

47 Frenk, J., Chen, L., Bhutta, Z. A., Cohen, J., Crisp, N., Evans, T., Fineberg, H., Garcia, P., Ke, Y., Kelley, P., Kistnasamy, B., Meleis, A., Naylor, D., Pablos-Mendez, A., Reddy, S., Scrimshaw, S., Sepulveda, J., Serwadda, D., & Zurayk, H. (2010). Health professionals for a new century: Transforming education to strengthen health systems in an interdependent world. *Lancet*, *376*(9756), 1923–1958. https://doi.org/10.1016/S0140-6736(10)61854-5

This paradigm was revisited after the pandemic[48] and serves as the basis for an expansive American Medical Association (AMA) project to transform medical education.[49,50] It further informs our discussion in this and subsequent chapters; its unique contribution is in pointing out that expertise can be routine with the practitioner in "autopilot" mode. This approach associated the adaptive expertise and master adaptive learner with professional identity formation (PIF) and attainment of mastery and phronesis, and may also be applied to systems through enlightened change agents.

AN OUNCE OF HUMILITY

Finally, we introduce **Trinh**'s study of "the curse of knowledge and cognitive entrenchment, which prevents [experts] from being able to adapt to changing situational demands."[51] This study was prompted by the collapse of corporations that were unable to cope with disruptive technology despite remarkable expertise in their respective domains (such as Nokia when smartphones appeared on the market). Trinh concludes:

> Acquiring and training experts to be able to quickly respond to the changing environments has been and will always be a big challenge for all organizations in this day and age. The solution sometimes may be counterintuitive: that one has to unlearn what one has learned, refrain from doing what has been successful, and keep in perspective what one has achieved. Having a piece of the humble pie and the mindset

48 Frenk, J., Chen, L. C., Chandran, L., Groff, E. O. H., King, R., Meleis, A., & Fineberg, H. V. (2022). Challenges and opportunities for educating health professionals after the COVID-19 pandemic. *Lancet*, *400*(10362), 1539–1556. https://doi .org/10.1016/S0140-6736(22)02092-X

49 Lomis, K. D., Santen, S. A., Dekhtyar, M., Elliott, V. S., Richardson, J., Hammoud, M. M., Hawkins, R., & Skochelak, S. E. (2021). The accelerating change in medical education consortium: Key drivers of transformative change. *Academic Medicine: Journal of the Association of American Medical Colleges*, *96*(7), 979–988. https:// doi.org/10.1097/ACM.0000000000003897

50 Skochelak, S. E., Lomis, K. D., Andrews, J. S., Hammoud, M. M., Mejicano, G. C., & Byerley, J. (2021). Realizing the vision of the Lancet Commission on education of health professionals for the 21st century: Transforming medical education through the accelerating change in medical education consortium. *Medical Teacher*, *43*(Suppl 2), S1–S6. https://doi.org/10.1080/0142159X.2021.1935833

51 Trinh, M. P. (2019). Overcoming the shadow of expertise: How humility and learning goal orientation help knowledge leaders become more flexible. *Frontiers in Psychology*, *10*, 2505. https://doi.org/10.3389/fpsyg.2019.02505

to continually learn new practices will help our knowledge experts go farther and be more resilient in today's uncertain world.

Summary

Although they may be unaware of it, the physicians in this chapter's opening story embody their metacognitive acumen. This category offers a transition to the constructs of expertise, mastery, and phronesis as goals of physician clinical reasoning and performance. Extending beyond the informative level, it also adds the formative and transformative as learning level goals. The expertise development literature includes an additional developmental stage model and innovates by pointing to pursuing the best possible performance rather than settling for "good enough." It identifies a correlation between reflective capacity (expanded upon in Chapter 5) and clinical reasoning, and proposes a framework for how the evolving physician uses deliberate practice to become a fully-fledged master adaptive expert. In addition, this category also highlights the ZPD nature of developmental spaces (another allusion to liminality), with Engeström expanding the ZPD to apply to collective expertise as well. Further, the informative–formative–transformative paradigm enables the integration and synergy of the various constructs. Finally, while this category introduces metacognition and intuition as valid constructs for expertise development, it also calls for "an ounce of humility."

The first three categories resonate with each other and readily find their place within PIF and the final, integrated understanding of the doctor's life cycle (DLC). It becomes clear that stages of development are not linear and continuous, but rather transformational nodes. A transition is an event that, once crossed, leads to a next level that is qualitatively distinct with its new comfort zone and zone of proximal development. These stages highlight that while the potential and frameworks for maximizing the doctor's potential exist, most physicians do not reach their full potential. Can this be modified? As in the first two categories, this category also ignores the adverse impact of gender- and race-related discrimination, as well as the DLC in the developing world, on expertise and phronesis. We address these aspects in Chapters 6–8.

REFERENCES

Betinol, E., Murphy, S., & Regehr, G. (2023). Exploring the development of adaptive expertise through the lens of threshold concepts. *Medical Education*, *57*(2), 142–150. https://doi.org/10.1111/medu.14887

Carraccio, C. L., Benson, B. J., Nixon, L. J., & Derstine, P. L. (2008). From the educational bench to the clinical bedside: Translating the Dreyfus developmental model to the learning of clinical skills. *Academic Medicine: Journal of the Association of American Medical Colleges, 83*(8), 761–767. https://doi.org/10.1097/ACM.0b013e31817eb632

Causer, J., Barach, P., & Williams, A. M. (2014). Expertise in medicine: Using the expert performance approach to improve simulation training. *Medical Education, 48*(2), 115–123. https://doi.org/10.1111/medu.12306

Cosgrove, L., & Shaughnessy, A. F. (2023). Becoming a phronimos: Evidence-based medicine, clinical decision making, and the role of practical wisdom in primary care. *Journal of the American Board of Family Medicine: JABFM, 36*(4), 531–536. https://doi.org/10.3122/jabfm.2023.230034R1

Cutrer, W. B., Miller, B., Pusic, M. V., Mejicano, G., Mangrulkar, R. S., Gruppen, L. D., Hawkins, R. E., Skochelak, S. E., & Moore, D. E., Jr. (2017). Fostering the development of master adaptive learners: A conceptual model to guide skill acquisition in medical education. *Academic Medicine: Journal of the Association of American Medical Colleges, 92*(1), 70–75. https://doi.org/10.1097/ACM.0000000000001323

Dearani, J. A., Gold, M., Leibovich, B. C., Ericsson, K. A., Khabbaz, K. R., Foley, T. A., Julsrud, P. R., Matsumoto, J. M., & Daly, R. C. (2017). The role of imaging, deliberate practice, structure, and improvisation in approaching surgical perfection. *Journal of Thoracic and Cardiovascular Surgery, 154*(4), 1329–1336. https://doi.org/10.1016/j.jtcvs.2017.04.045

Dreyfus, H. (2006, September 9). *From novice to world discloser.* Paper presented at the Accreditation Council for Graduate Medical Education Design Conference on the Learning Environment, Chicago, IL.

Dreyfus, H., & Dreyfus, S. E. (1987). *Mind over machine: The power of human intuition and expertise in the era of the computer.* Free Press.

Durning, S. J., Costanzo, M. E., Beckman, T. J., Artino, A. R., Jr, Roy, M. J., van der Vleuten, C., Holmboe, E. S., Lipner, R. S., & Schuwirth, L. (2016). Functional neuroimaging correlates of thinking flexibility and knowledge structure in memory: Exploring the relationships between clinical reasoning and diagnostic thinking. *Medical Teacher, 38*(6), 570–577. https://doi.org/10.3109/0142159X.2015.1047755

Engeström, Y. (2018). *Expertise in transition: Expansive learning in medical work.* Cambridge University Press. https://doi.org/10.1017/9781139023009

Ericsson, K. A. (2015). Acquisition and maintenance of medical expertise: A perspective from the expert-performance approach with deliberate practice. *Academic Medicine: Journal of the Association of American Medical Colleges, 90*(11), 1471–1486. https://doi.org/10.1097/ACM.0000000000000939

Ericsson, K. A., & Harwell, K. W. (2019). Deliberate practice and proposed limits on the effects of practice on the acquisition of expert performance: Why the original definition matters and recommendations for future research. *Frontiers in Psychology, 10*, 2396. https://doi.org/10.3389/fpsyg.2019.02396

Ericsson, K. A., Hoffman, R. R., Kozbelt, A., & Williams, A. M. (Eds.). (2018). *The Cambridge handbook of expertise and expert performance* (2nd ed.). Cambridge University Press. https://doi.org/10.1017/9781316480748

Ericsson, K. A., Nandagopal, K., & Roring, R. W. (2009). Toward a science of exceptional achievement: Attaining superior performance through deliberate practice. *Annals of the New York Academy of Sciences, 1172*, 199–217. https://doi.org/10.1196/annals.1393.001

Ericsson, K. A., & Pool, R. (2016). *Peak: How all of us can achieve extraordinary things.* Vintage.

Frank, A. W. (2012). Reflective healthcare practice: Claims, phronesis and dialogue. In E. A. Kinsella & A. Pitman (Eds.), *Phronesis as professional knowledge: Practical wisdom in the professions* (pp. 53–60). Sense Publishers. https://doi.org/10.1007 /978-94-6091-731-8

Frenk, J., Chen, L. C., Bhutta, Z. A., Cohen, J., Crisp, N., Evans, T., Fineberg, H., Garcia, P., Ke, Y., Kelley, P., Kistnasamy, B., Meleis, A., Naylor, D., Pablos-Mendez, A., Reddy, S., Scrimshaw, S., Sepulveda, J., Serwadda, D., & Zurayk, H. (2010). Health professionals for a new century: Transforming education to strengthen health systems in an interdependent world. *Lancet, 376*(9756), 1923–1958. https:// doi.org/10.1016/S0140-6736(10)61854-5

Frenk, J., Chen, L. C., Chandran, L., Groff, E. O. H., King, R., Meleis, A., & Fineberg, H. V. (2022). Challenges and opportunities for educating health professionals after the COVID-19 pandemic. *Lancet, 400*(10362), 1539–1556. https://doi.org/10.1016 /S0140-6736(22)02092-X

Gladwell, M. (2008). *Outliers: The story of success.* Little, Brown and Company.

Groopman, J. (2007). *How doctors think.* Houghton Mifflin.

Groot, F., Jonker, G., Rinia, M., Ten Cate, O., & Hoff, R. G. (2020). Simulation at the frontier of the zone of proximal development: A test in acute care for inexperienced learners. *Academic Medicine: Journal of the Association of American Medical Colleges, 95*(7), 1098–1105. https://doi.org/10.1097/ACM.0000000000003265

Hastings, R. H., & Rickard, T. C. (2015). Deliberate practice for achieving and maintaining expertise in anesthesiology. *Anesthesia and Analgesia, 120*(2), 449–459. https://doi.org/10.1213/ANE.0000000000000526

Kinsella, E. A., & Pitman, A. (Eds.). (2012). *Phronesis as professional knowledge: Practical wisdom in the professions.* Sense Publishers. https://doi.org/10.1007/978 -94-6091-731-8

Krackov, S. K., & Pohl, H. (2011). Building expertise using the deliberate practice curriculum-planning model. *Medical Teacher, 33*(7), 570–575. https://doi.org/10 .3109/0142159X.2011.578172

Kumagai, A. K. (2022). Discomfort, doubt, and the edge of learning. *Academic Medicine: Journal of the Association of American Medical Colleges, 97*(5), 649–654. https:// doi.org/10.1097/ACM.0000000000004588

Li, Q., Wang, X., Wang, S., Xie, Y., Li, X., Xie, Y., & Li, S. (2019). Dynamic reconfiguration of the functional brain network after musical training in young adults. *Brain Structure & Function, 224*(5), 1781–1795. https://doi.org/10.1007/ s00429-019-01867-z

Lomis, K. D., Santen, S. A., Dekhtyar, M., Elliott, V. S., Richardson, J., Hammoud, M. M., Hawkins, R., & Skochelak, S. E. (2021). The accelerating change in medical education consortium: Key drivers of transformative change. *Academic Medicine: Journal of the Association of American Medical Colleges, 96*(7), 979–988. https:// doi.org/10.1097/ACM.0000000000003897

Mamede, S., Figueiredo-Soares, T., Elói Santos, S. M., de Faria, R. M. D., Schmidt, H. G., & van Gog, T. (2019). Fostering novice students' diagnostic ability: The value of guiding deliberate reflection. *Medical Education, 53*(6), 628–637. https://doi.org /10.1111/medu.13829

Mamede, S., Hautz, W. E., Berendonk, C., Hautz, S. C., Sauter, T. C., Rotgans, J., Zwaan, L., & Schmidt, H. G. (2020). Think twice: Effects on diagnostic accuracy of returning to the case to reflect upon the initial diagnosis. *Academic Medicine: Journal of the Association of American Medical Colleges, 95*(8), 1223–1229. https://doi.org/10.1097/ACM.0000000000003153

Mamede, S., & Schmidt, H. G. (2004). The structure of reflective practice in medicine. *Medical Education, 38*(12), 1302–1308. https://doi.org/10.1111/j.1365-2929.2004 .01917.x

McGaghie, W. C., Issenberg, S. B., Cohen, E. R., Barsuk, J. H., & Wayne, D. B. (2011). Does simulation-based medical education with deliberate practice yield better results than traditional clinical education? A meta-analytic comparative review of the evidence. *Academic Medicine: Journal of the Association of American Medical Colleges*, 86(6), 706–711. https://doi.org/10.1097/ACM.0b013e318217e119

Montgomery, K. (2006). *How doctors think: Clinical judgment and the practice of medicine*. Oxford University Press.

Paes, P. (2019). Practical wisdom, a dormant character in medical education? *Medical Education*, 53(5), 428–429. https://doi.org/10.1111/medu.13832

Paes, P., Leat, D., & Stewart, J. (2019). Complex decision making in medical training: Key internal and external influences in developing practical wisdom. *Medical Education*, 53(2), 165–174. https://doi.org/10.1111/medu.13767

Petty, T. L. (1979). Don't just do something—stand there! *Archives of Internal Medicine*, 139(8), 920–921. https://doi.org/10.1001/archinte.1979.03630450062020

Quirk, M. (2006). *Intuition and metacognition in medical education: Keys to developing expertise*. Springer.

Reis, S., & Klein, M. (2011). Such naches. *Patient Education and Counseling*, 83, 45–46. https://doi.org/10.1016/j.pec.2010.03.012

Rissmiller, B., Castro, D., Minard, C. G., Sur, M., Roy, K., Turner, T., & Thammasitboon, S. (2019). The diagnostic expertise acceleration module (DEAM): Promoting the formation of organized knowledge. *Medical Education Online*, 24(1). https://doi.org/10.1080/10872981.2019.1679945

Sandars, J., Allan, D., & Price, J. (2023). Reflective practice by health professions educators to enhance learning and teaching: AMEE Guide No. 166. *Medical Teacher*, 1–10. https://doi.org/10.1080/0142159X.2023.2259071

Schei, E., Knoop, H. S., Gismervik, M. N., Mylopoulos, M., & Boudreau, J. D. (2019). Stretching the comfort zone: Using early clinical contact to influence professional identity formation in medical students. *Journal of Medical Education and Curricular Development*, 6. https://doi.org/10.1177/2382120519843875

Schmidt, H. G., Norman, G. R., & Boshuizen, H. P. (1990). A cognitive perspective on medical expertise: Theory and implication. *Academic Medicine: Journal of the Association of American Medical Colleges*, 65(10), 611–621. https://doi.org/10.1097/00001888-199010000-00001

Schmidt, P. C., & Fenner, D. E. (2020). Deliberate practice: Applying the expert performance approach to gynecologic surgical training. *Clinical Obstetrics and Gynecology*, 63(2), 295–304. https://doi.org/10.1097/GRF.0000000000000509

Shachak, A., Buchanan, F., & Kuziemsky, C. (2024). When rules turn into tools: An activity theory-based perspective on implementation processes and unintended consequences. *Healthcare Management Forum*, 37(3), 177–182. https://doi.org/10.1177/08404704241233169

Shah, A. P., Walker, K. A., Hawick, L., Walker, K. G., & Cleland, J. (2023). Scratching beneath the surface: How organisational culture influences curricular reform. *Medical Education*, 57(7), 668–678. https://doi.org/10.1111/medu.14994

Skochelak, S. E., Lomis, K. D., Andrews, J. S., Hammoud, M. M., Mejicano, G. C., & Byerley, J. (2021). Realizing the vision of the Lancet Commission on education of health professionals for the 21st century: Transforming medical education through the accelerating change in medical education consortium. *Medical Teacher*, 43(Suppl 2), S1–S6. https://doi.org/10.1080/0142159X.2021.1935833

Trinh, M. P. (2019). Overcoming the shadow of expertise: How humility and learning goal orientation help knowledge leaders become more flexible. *Frontiers in Psychology*, 10, 2505. https://doi.org/10.3389/fpsyg.2019.02505

Waite, S., Farooq, Z., Grigorian, A., Sistrom, C., Kolla, S., Mancuso, A., Martinez-Conde, S., Alexander, R. G., Kantor, A., & Macknik, S. L. (2020). A review of perceptual expertise in radiology-How it develops, how we can test it, and why humans still matter in the era of artificial intelligence. *Academic Radiology*, 27(1), 26–38. https://doi.org/10.1016/j.acra.2019.08.018

CHAPTER 4

Moral and character development

....

What is going on in Ukraine will change us forever

Challenging images are emerging from Ukraine. Dozens of babies whisked from the newborn nursery, out of harm's way, into a makeshift basement shelter snuggled together for warmth. An adult gently, manually "Ambu-bags" a tiny person who should be on a mechanical ventilator. Lines, miles long, of the elderly, women, and children on the move. These images don't only generate horror and deep empathy for the immediate danger and distress: for many of us, even if we never personally, directly experienced that level of terror, loss, or permanent displacement, bitter memories emerge.

For me—and based on my own family's experiences—my empathy is built on an intimate knowledge of the very long road ahead for those lucky enough to survive. Trauma of this level reverberates down the years, not only because of the deaths and destruction of places and cultures, but because of the inexorable impact on the health and wellbeing of the survivors and the following generations.

Refugee crises have occurred with great regularity, sometimes due to natural events, but usually as the result of the aggression of despotic national leaders and their enablers. This mass migration of Ukrainians is likely to rival, in speed and size, that resulting from the Balkan War in the early 1990s and lead to—if this conflict lasts much longer—the displacement of several million persons, with suffering not seen since the 1940s. Based on history, we can predict the short- and long-term

DOI: 10.1201/9781003507529-5

impact of this crisis, and it is not a pretty picture. If we are seriously committed to human health, wellbeing, and flourishing, we need to act now.

My mother was a refugee

In September 1939, when my mother was only three years old, the German Army invaded her country. A few weeks later, the family wrapped a set of silver candlesticks, a photo album, and a few other items in a blanket and—hiding in a hay wagon—followed the retreating Polish Army east from their town of Suwalki into Russia. They left everything, everyone, and their large, vibrant family behind. In retrospect, they considered themselves very lucky to have been able to live out the war in a work settlement in Murmansk, Russia, despite periodic aerial bombardment by the German Army. They were grateful to be relatively safe although, sometimes, they had neither enough food nor any news from their loved ones.

This week, Ukrainian families, including many children, are sleeping in deep subterranean subway stations and underground parking lots. Parents are telling their little ones stories—like my grandparents told my mother—hoping to transform the loud noises into an adventure. But the children, no doubt, feel terror and see the adults arming themselves.

Stark, full-color, high-definition images show men and women in civilian clothes working in bunkers, rifles slung over the shoulders, and filling beer bottles to create Molotov cocktails. These are people who, only days before, were living peaceful lives, working desk jobs, and going to shopping malls. Life turned on a dime. Yesterday, you were a salesclerk in a department store and today you are making a "poor man's grenade" to throw at tanks rolling down a street in your home city. Unthinkable.

The cataclysmic transformation in their lives brought a flood of entirely unearned grainy black and white memories, unearned because they are not directly mine but an intergenerational inheritance.

After the war, my mother and her parents made their way to a displaced persons camp in US-occupied, demilitarized Munich, Germany, where they were reunited with what was left of their family. After two years, they sailed, in steerage, to Galveston, Texas, where they had relatives, and were relocated by HIAS (the Hebrew Immigrant Aid Society)—which was established in 1881 and is still very active in advocacy, directly serving refugees and immigrants from around the world—to Vineland, New Jersey. There, as urban-dwelling, small business owners, they lived together and tried (unsuccessfully) to run a chicken farm.

My mother was the salutatorian of her high school class less than four years after arriving in the United States. When she arrived, she spoke three languages (Yiddish, Polish, Russian) and learned English and some Spanish soon after. As the second youngest in the family (a cousin was born in the displaced persons camp), she adapted quickly and was often the one who facilitated the intercultural communication between the family and the Americans.

I often thought of my mother when I was seeing immigrant families in my primary care clinic. It was common that adults brought along their youngsters who would advocate, translate, and culturally interpret for their adult relatives. This is problematic, as you can imagine, in so many ways. Not the least of which is those kids were not in school! But this was a role my mother played, with devotion and pride, her whole life.

Why am I telling this story?

Trauma leads to shortened lives filled with disabling physical and emotional consequences. My grandfather died of a heart attack at fifty-four. My mother's cousins, who had survived into young adulthood as partisan fighters or in concentration camps, struggled with lifelong health issues. One cousin had a heart attack in his early thirties, another underwent many surgeries to repair the damage caused by a land mine. Heart disease was ubiquitous. I grew up thinking it was normal that toward the end of a large holiday meal, one of the adults would need to be escorted into the bedroom for supplemental oxygen and intravenous diuresis. I flash back to the image of my grandmother, then only a few years older than I am now, slowly walking up our sidewalk, her edematous ankles spilling over the edge of her flat, utilitarian "old lady" shoes.

My mother, who lived most of her life peacefully and happily in America, died, suddenly and unexpectedly, at fifty-five from complications of a heart attack. While this was over forty years after she emigrated, there is no doubt that her early war- and displacement-based life experiences led to this premature death and, therefore, she never met her grandchildren. An incalculable loss.

The personal and biologic effects of displacement

For many years, even given my extensive medical and public health education, I thought the family curse of early heart disease was almost entirely genetic and, therefore, unavoidable. I follow with great interest (for myself, my sibling, and our children) the work on epigenetics which suggests that the children of survivors of trauma biologically inherit a tendency toward chronic elevation of stress hormones. Researchers have demonstrated that the allostatic load—or the wear and tear on the body—accumulates under repeated or chronic stress, leading to fluctuations in neuroendocrine responses, as well as changes in cortisol and catecholamine levels, which significantly increases the risk of cardiovascular disease and death from all causes.

People suffer when their lives are disrupted, either chronically (as in racism) or acutely (as in war). We know a bit more about how we can reduce and interrupt the negative impact, by working with individuals, at the community level, and with public policy. I now understand, as is supported by science, that there are trauma-informed ways to address or reverse the life consequences of chronic fear, constant vigilance, and stress on our bodies. Unfortunately, we will need to keep ramping up these efforts.

After my mother's death, my father and I went to talk to her physician. He had seen her a couple of days before she died and talked about his sadness and regret that he had "missed" the seriousness of her situation. My mother was unlikely to complain or draw attention to herself. "She talked about her discomfort as if it were happening to someone else." This threw him off, even knowing the emerging research that women's myocardial infarctions can present (as she had described) with upper abdomen rather than left chest pain, and knowing that physicians tend to underdiagnose significant coronary heart disease in women for a myriad of reasons. I was not surprised to hear this.

My mother was stoic and preternaturally calm by nature and nurture. While I have long since forgiven him for this misjudgment, I couldn't help but think that if he had known her better and had understood her life story, he might have been more attuned to her distress. She might have used those candlesticks for many more Sabbaths. She might have met her grandchildren.

Ultimately, the best way to address the adverse intergenerational legacy of war is to insist on peace. In the meantime, offering real, meaningful care and compassion for those in immediate need matters a great deal and saves lives.

The resolve of Ukrainian resistance has apparently surprised the Russian invaders and inspired us all. NATO countries and allies' severe financial sanctions are having their intended impacts. Facebook and Twitter have dampened noxious misinformation and stopped bots from interfering with critical infrastructure, and large antiwar protests are taking place around the world, including in Russia.

The future is very uncertain, and the situation is, as it should be, very frightening. More is needed now. There are too many people being forced to take a journey reminiscent of the one my mother and her family were forced to take. That hay cart forever led them away from their home, their extended family, and the chance of living a long and healthy life.[1]

* * *

Kalet's World War II family refugee story and her reflection on Russia's invasion of Ukraine are sobering reminders of how war disrupts lives for generations to come. It is also an alarming wake-up call alerting us that

---

1   Kalet, A. (2022, April 22). What is going on in Ukraine will change us forever. *Transformational Times: Newsletter of the Robert D. and Patricia E. Kern Institute for the Transformation of Medical Education.*

war crimes, crimes against humanity, human rights violations, and mass atrocities are still occurring in the heart of Europe almost 80 years after these constructs were created to persecute Nazi perpetrators. Physicians and medicine were responsible for heinous Nazi medical crimes during the Holocaust, the genocide of European Jews.[2] Moreover, while this book was in its final stages of editing, Hamas massacred 1,200 civilians in southern Israel on October 7, 2023, and the war in Gaza ensued and is still ongoing. Millions of people in Gaza and hundreds of thousands in Israel are displaced.[3] The plight of civilians in Gaza is excruciating. Like in Ukraine, these massive displacements inevitably exert their noxious impact. In addition, the collusion of health professionals and the healthcare infrastructure in Gaza with terrorism raises grave concerns. Recently, a plea has been made to integrate into the medical ethos the detection, prevention, care, and rehabilitation of war crimes, mass atrocities, crimes against humanity, and genocide. This is a distressing prelude to the current state of humanity and healthcare, as well as to a discussion of physician moral development.

PHYSICIAN MORAL DEVELOPMENT

Moral and ethical conduct stands out as a fundamental competency that lends itself to maturation and development.[4] Some scholars see it as the most authentic proxy of medical professionalism. Instruction in medical and clinical ethics is proliferating[5,6] and attention is being paid

2   Czech, H., Hildebrandt, S., Reis, S. P., Chelouche, T., Fox, M., González-López, E., Lepicard, E., Ley, A., Offer, M., Ohry, A., Rotzoll, M., Sachse, C., Siegel, S. J., Šimůnek, M., Teicher, A., Uzarczyk, K., von Villiez, A., Wald, H. S., Wynia, M. K., & Roelcke, V. (2023). The Lancet Commission on medicine, Nazism, and the Holocaust: Historical evidence, implications for today, teaching for tomorrow. *Lancet*, *402*(10415), 1867–1940. https://doi.org/10.1016/S0140-6736(23)01845-7

3   Reis, S. P., & Wald, H. S. (2024). The Hamas massacre of Oct 7, 2023, and its aftermath, medical crimes, and the Lancet Commission report on medicine, Nazism, and the Holocaust. *Israel Journal of Health Policy Research*, *13*(1), 19. https://doi.org/10.1186/s13584-024-00608-w

4   Rest, J. R. (1993). Research on moral judgment in college students. In A. Garrod (Ed.), *Approaches to moral development: New research and emerging themes* (pp. 201–213). Teachers College Press.

5   Jakubowski, H., Xie, J., Kumar Mitra, A., Ghooi, R., Hosseinkhani, S., Alipour, M., Hajipour, B., & Obiero, G. (2017). The global ethics corner: Foundations, beliefs, and the teaching of biomedical and scientific ethics around the world. *Biochemistry and Molecular Biology Education: A Bimonthly Publication of the International Union of Biochemistry and Molecular Biology*, *45*(5), 385–395. https://doi.org/10.1002/bmb.21059

6   Brooks, L., & Bell, D. (2017). Teaching, learning and assessment of medical ethics at the UK medical schools. *Journal of Medical Ethics*, *43*(9), 606–612. https://doi.org/10.1136/medethics-2015-103189

to non-cognitive attributes, morality included, in both medical school admissions and assessment. Accordingly, the core constructs of this fourth category include moral development, as well as moral distress[7] and moral injury,[8] which are relatively new concepts in medical education. A few researchers in this domain closely associate the construct of character development with moral development.[9,10]

Following **Piaget**'s groundbreaking work on moral judgment in children, **Kohlberg** expanded the field of moral and developmental psychology.[11] Both used a "stage and sequence" paradigm (echoed in our first three categories), which has been subsequently criticized.[12] A theory of moral development was first postulated by Kohlberg (Figure 4.1) and subjected to rigorous research through the development of an assessment instrument, the Defining Issues Test (DIT). This work joins with other social cognitive stage models developed in the 1980s.

Kohlberg described three levels of moral development: **pre-conventional (early years), conventional (adolescence and adulthood),** and **postconventional (morally mature)**. Each level is subdivided into two stages, resulting in a six-stage model. Kohlberg's approach was challenged by feminist **Carol Gilligan**, who criticized his work for ignoring the care orientation and focusing exclusively on the justice orientation as the goal of moral development. Gilligan proposed her stage theory of female moral development based on her idea of moral voices, asserting that there are two moral voices or preferences: the masculine and the feminine. The masculine voice is "logical and individualistic," emphasizing moral decisions such as protecting the rights of people and ensuring that justice is upheld as paramount. The feminine voice places greater emphasis on

7   Waldman, R. A., Waldman, S. D., & Carter, B. S. (2019). When I say… moral distress as a teaching point. *Medical Education, 53*(5), 430–431. https://doi.org/10.1111/medu.13769

8   Ford, E. W. (2019). Stress, burnout, and moral injury: The state of the healthcare workforce. *Journal of Healthcare Management/American College of Healthcare Executives, 64*(3), 125–127. https://doi.org/10.1097/JHM-D-19-00058

9   Bebeau, M. J. (2006). Evidence based character development. In N. P. Kenny & W. Shelton (Eds.), *Lost virtue: Professional character development in medical education. Advances in Bioethics 10,* 47–86. https://doi.org/10.1016/S1479-3709(06)10004-7

10 Bryan, C. S., & Babelay, A. M. (2009). Building character: A model for reflective practice. *Academic Medicine: Journal of the Association of American Medical Colleges, 84*(9), 1283–1288. https://doi.org/10.1097/ACM.0b013e3181b6a79c

11 Rest, J. R., Thoma, S. J., & Edwards, L. (1997). Designing and validating a measure of moral judgment: Stage preference and stage consistency approaches. *Journal of Educational Psychology 89*(1), 5–28. https://doi.org/10.1037/0022-0663.89.1.5

12 Gilligan, C. (1982). *In a different voice: Psychological theory and women's development.* Harvard University Press.

Kohlberg's Theory of Moral Development

Level 3	Post-conventional	• **Stage 6:** Self-selecting universal principles
		• **Stage 5:** Sensing the democracy and relativity of rules
Level 2	Conventional	• **Stage 4:** Fulfilling duties and upholding laws
		• **Stage 3:** Meeting the expectations of others
Level 1	Pre-conventional	• **Stage 2:** "Getting what you want" by reciprocity
		• **Stage 1:** Avoiding punishment

FIGURE 4.1 Kohlberg's Stages of Moral Development. (Public domain.)

protecting interpersonal relationships and taking care of others. This voice is the "care perspective," where one focuses on the needs of the individual in order to make an ethical decision.

For Gilligan, Kohlberg's stages of moral development emphasize the masculine voice, making it difficult to accurately gauge and value the care perspective of human moral development in both men and women. Gilligan argues that "integrating the masculine and the feminine, is the best way to realize one's potential as a human." This criticism led to the development of a neo-Kohlbergian model, also known as **Rest's Four Component Model (FCM)**,[13] which incorporates aspects of schema theory (cognitive psychology, introduced in Chapter 3) and directly addresses post-conventional (adult) moral development. This model describes four human capacities needed for consistent moral behavior: **moral/ethical sensitivity, moral judgment/reasoning, moral motivation/commitment, and moral action/character.** Within the judgment/reasoning capacity, scholars have identified the constructs of **codes of conduct, intermediate concepts, and bedrock schema**, postulating them as the basis for **profession-specific reasoning**.[14]

---

13 Rest, J., Narvaez, D., Bebeau, M., & Thoma, S. (1999). A neo-Kohlbergian approach: The DIT and schema theory. *Educational Psychology Review, 11*(4), 291–324. https://doi.org/10.1023/A:1022053215271

14 Bebeau, M. J., & Thoma, S. J. (1999). "Intermediate" concepts and the connection to moral education. *Educational Psychology Review, 11*(4), 343–360. https://psycnet.apa.org/doi/10.1023/A:1022057316180

MEASUREMENT OF MORAL DEVELOPMENT

Multiple instruments have been proposed to gauge the various levels and stages of moral and ethical development. The DIT-2[15,16,17,18,19,20] is the most widely used measure of individual capacity for judgment/reasoning based on moral principles. Yet, the four neo-Kohlbergian capacities are not perfect predictors of actual moral behavior. Medical education literature accepts that moral and ethical behaviors are context-dependent rather than reflections of stable personality traits[21] and that they may not lend themselves to a reliable and valid competence/performance measurement. Presently, no medicine-specific, valid, and reliable instrument exists, and researchers employ generic ones. However, the neo-Kohlbergian capacities and relevant measures such as the DIT-2 and Professional Identity Essay (PIE) have proven useful in conducting effective remediation for lapses in professionalism and in curriculum evaluation.[22]

MORAL AND CHARACTER DEVELOPMENT, AND THE VIRTUOUS PHYSICIAN

Scholars of moral development have considered moral, character, and identity development to be very closely related. For example, Bebeau writes:

15 Self, D. J., Baldwin, D. C., Jr., & Wolinsky, F. D. (1992). Evaluation of teaching medical ethics by an assessment of moral reasoning. *Medical Education*, 26(3), 178–184. https://doi.org/10.1111/j.1365-2923.1992.tb00151.x

16 Walker, L. J. (2002). The model and the measure: An appraisal of the Minnesota approach to moral development. *Journal of Moral Education*, 31(3), 353–367. https://doi.org/10.1080/0305724022000008160

17 Regehr, G. (2006). The persistent myth of stability. On the chronic underestimation of the role of context in behavior. *Journal of General Internal Medicine*, 21(5), 544–545. https://doi.org/10.1111/j.1525-1497.2006.00447.x

18 Bebeau, M. J. (2002). The defining issues test and the four-component model: Contributions to professional education. *Journal of Moral Education*, 31(3), 271–295. https://doi.org/10.1080/0305724022000008115

19 Monson, V., Bebeau, M. J., Faber-Langendoen, K., & Kalet, A. (2023). Professionalism lapses as professional identity formation challenges. In A. Kalet & C. L. Chou (Eds.), *Remediation in medical education* (pp. 147–161). Springer. https://doi.org/10.1007/978-3-031-32404-8_13

20 Bebeau, M. J., & Monson, V. E. (2012). Professional identity formation and transformation across the life span. In A. Mc Kee & M. Eraut (Eds.), *Learning trajectories, innovation and identity for professional development* (pp. 135–162). Springer. https://doi.org/10.1007/978-94-007-1724-4_7

21 Patenaude, J., Niyonsenga, T., & Fafard, D. (2003). Changes in the components of moral reasoning during students' medical education: A pilot study. *Medical Education*, 37(9), 822–829. https://doi.org/10.1046/j.1365-2923.2003.01593.x

22 Baldwin, D. C., Jr., Daugherty, S., & Self, D. J. (1991). Changes in moral reasoning during medical school. *Academic Medicine: Journal of the Association of American Medical Colleges*, 66(Suppl 9), S1, 1–3.

> Briefly stated, individuals move from self-centered conceptions of identity through a number of transitions, to a moral identity characterized by the expectations of a "profession" – to put the interests of others before the self. … The fully integrated moral self (one whose personal and professional values are fully integrated and consistently applied) tends not to develop until midlife – if it develops at all.

This sentiment resonates with the previous category, which observed that most physicians may not reach their full potential or expertise and mastery. Understanding how the individual conceptualizes the self in relation to others provides valuable insights into lapses in ethical behavior, especially in instances where the moral choice is well understood.[23,24,25]

Bebeau was assigned the assessment and remediation of dental practitioners in Minnesota, USA, who were brought before a disciplinary board to regain their dental license.[26,27] She describes an elaborate process of preparatory work, a diagnostic half day (in which five validated instruments are filled out by the remediating practitioner), discussion of the findings, drafting a plan, and evaluating its success so that a license can be regranted. Forty-one individuals are described in her 2009 papers. Similar programs exist for physicians in the United Kingdom, Australia, and the United States.

Bebeau reviews the evidence concerning the development of ethical decision-making competencies in medical professionals. She examines selected studies that use a theoretical framework, which shows the most promise for providing evidence of character formation. The findings suggest that entering professionals lack the full capacity for functional processes that give rise to morality, such as sensitivity, reasoning, motivation

23 Thaxton, R. E., Jones, W. S., Hafferty, F. W., April, C. W., & April, M. D. (2018). Self vs. other focus: Predicting professionalism remediation of emergency medicine residents. *Western Journal of Emergency Medicine*, 19(1), 35–40. https://doi.org/10.5811/westjem.2017.11.35242

24 Lessing, J. N., Bryan, S., Johnson, C., Keating, J., & Guerrasio, J. (2019). Junior doctor remediation: An international reflection. *Medical Journal of Australia*, 211(11), 507–508.e1. https://doi.org/10.5694/mja2.50422

25 Skelton, J. R., Wiskin, C. M., & Ward, J. D. T. (2019). Understanding professional development: Case studies of remedial support. *Medical Teacher*, 41(12), 1372–1379. https://doi.org/10.1080/0142159X.2019.1638896

26 Bebeau, M. J. (2009). Enhancing professionalism using ethics education as part of a dental licensure board's disciplinary action. Part 1. An evidence-based process. *Journal of the American College of Dentists*, 76(2), 38–50.

27 Bebeau M. J. (2009). Enhancing professionalism using ethics education as part of a dental licensure board's disciplinary action. Part 2. Evidence of the process. *Journal of the American College of Dentists*, 76(3), 32–45.

and commitment, character, and competence. Bebeau concludes with suggestions for facilitating character development resistant to influence by negative role models or adverse moral milieus.

Further research indicates that considerable variations in moral abilities also persist following professional education. Whereas many perceive that role modeling is the most effective way to teach professionalism and morality, instruction on the cognitive basis of professionalism is also needed.

Fatima,[28] **Hawking** et al.,[29] and **Kotzee** and **Ignatowicz**[30] argue that conventional moral development scholars are focused on **moral reasoning,** while **moral behavior** stems from a nexus of **intuitive moral emotions.** Subsequently joined by cognitive morality, these components constitute optional virtuous conduct. To these authors, **virtue ethics** is based on character, and other authors recommend its incorporation in professional identity formation (PIF), mentioning courage as an attribute of the virtuous physician, along with empathy, compassion, and wisdom.[31] Hawking et al. identify "difficult" patients as the "moral stress test" and suggest pedagogies to enhance the **formation of physicians of virtuous character.**

LIVING A MORAL LIFE IN MEDICINE: THE MORAL IDEAL–MORAL REALITY GAP

Kleinman, in his concern with living a moral life,[32] stresses that:

> A passion for doubting is a requirement of a moral life because we need to bring an aspiration for ethics to bear on moral experience. … What a lifetime of being with others in the messiness of moral experience has taught me is that simplistic distinctions between the objective and the subjective, the absolute and the relative, the right and the wrong, are no

28 Fatima, S. (2016). Can doctors maintain good character? An examination of physician lives. *Journal of Medical Humanities*, 37(4), 419–433. https://doi.org/10.1007/s10912-016-9385-5

29 Hawking, M., Curlin, F. A., & Yoon, J. D. (2017). Courage and compassion: Virtues in caring for so-called "difficult" patients. *AMA Journal of Ethics*, 19(4), 357–363. https://doi.org/10.1001/journalofethics.2017.19.4.medu2-1704

30 Kotzee, B., & Ignatowicz, A. (2016). Measuring 'virtue' in medicine. *Medicine, Health Care, and Philosophy*, 19(2), 149–161. https://doi.org/10.1007/s11019-015-9653-6

31 Kim, D. T., Applewhite, M. K., & Shelton, W. (2023). Professional identity formation in medical education: Some virtue-based insights. *Teaching and Learning in Medicine*, 1–11. Advance online publication. https://doi.org/10.1080/10401334.2023.2209067

32 Kleinman, A. (2006). *What really matters: Living a moral life amidst uncertainty and danger* (1st ed.). Oxford University Press.

help and may even get us into deeper trouble. … We must see moral experience for what it is: all that we have and all that we will ever have that defines our humanity and makes us and our worlds real. … Medical students learn to open one eye to the pain and suffering of patients and the world, but also to close the other eye—to protect their own vulnerability to pain and suffering, to protect their belief that they can do good and change the world for the better.

He points out that in this messy reality, all healers experience a **gap between a moral ideal and the daily moral experience**. Thus, **moral distress** and even injury become part of the professional's practice and life.[33] Moral distress is ubiquitous and may occur daily with instances of uncertainty, value conflicts, and the need to solve problems and make decisions, often under great pressure of need, time, and resources.

Additionally, in the hierarchical nature of medicine, superiors often give "orders" to their subordinates, which may create moral distress in their implementation. Kleinman describes moments of moral distress that may injure, morally, those who experience them. Psychiatrists diagnose such injury in practitioners who have encountered extreme situations such as combat and suggest that it may be common in healthcare: "Moral injury … occurs when someone must commit or witness an act that violates their moral belief system." Presently, students and practitioners are offered little support in weathering their moral experiences, distresses, and potential injuries, which may have profound effects on resilience, wellbeing, and performance, as well as on identity and character formation. The concepts of moral experience, distress, and injury move beyond the moral development literature and point to a complex and nuanced reality.

In his recent book,[34] as well as several earlier papers,[35,36,37] Kleinman takes his view on moral experience a step further by calling to move

33 Mollnaro, M. L., Shen, K., Agarwal, G., Inglis, G., & Vanstone, M. (2023). Family physicians' moral distress when caring for patients experiencing social inequities: A critical narrative inquiry in primary care. *British Journal of General Practice: The Journal of the Royal College of General Practitioners*, 74(738), e41–e48. https://doi .org/10.3399/BJGP.2023.0193

34 Kleinman, A. (2019). *The soul of care: moral education of a husband and doctor.* Viking.

35 Kleinman, A. (2016). Caring for memories. *Lancet*, 387(10038), 2596–2597. https:// doi.org/10.1016/s0140-6736(16)30853-4

36 Kleinman, A. (2014). How we endure. *Lancet*, 383(9912), 119–120. https://doi.org /10.1016/s0140-6736(14)60012-x

37 Kleinman, A. (2013). From illness as culture to caregiving as moral experience. *New England Journal of Medicine*, 368(15), 1376–1377. https://doi.org/10.1056/ NEJMp1300678

"from illness as culture to caregiving as moral experience." He describes how being a caregiver to his late wife, who contracted a devastating degenerative neurological disorder, "clarified the moral processes central to caregiving" and that "how to revivify caregiving in medicine became the issue." He asserts:

> Modern medical practice's greatest challenge may be finding a way to keep caregiving central to health care. That way will turn on … the importance that professionals ascribe to patients' deep experiences and to such enduring moral practices of caring as the laying on of hands, the expression of kindness, the enactment of decency, and the commitment to presence – being there for those who need them. This is the embodied wisdom medical students need to learn and we all must remember.

BEYOND PRINCIPLED ETHICS

Albeit complex, the basic stage model of moral development—which espouses the paradigm of principled ethics (justice, autonomy, beneficence, and non-maleficence)[38] that informs almost all ethics education and deliberation—once again encounters critics who point out that the lived moral experiences of learners and practitioners are nuanced and narrative by nature. There is an inherent gap between moral ideals and moral experiences in which principled ethics provides little guidance. Consequently, practitioners are left to face a personal, often hidden struggle of living a moral life involving imperfection, uncertainty, conflicting values, and sometimes error and failure. A life wherein witnessing and forgiving both oneself and others are essential.

Thus, immersion in this category fosters a need to find ways to reconcile principled ethics, virtue ethics, and character development with the real-life gap between the moral ideal and moral experience (the narrative ethics approach). Kleinman proposes that this may be achieved by keeping practical, hands-on caregiving central to both healthcare and health professions education. His "embodied wisdom" of caregiving seems aligned with the "practical wisdom" of expertise, further explored in the next category, where embodiment as part of personal and professional development is discussed. Kleinman's proposition also resonates with Gilligan's aforementioned feminine moral care orientation.

---

38 Beauchamp, T. L., & Childress, J. F. (2001). *Principles of biomedical ethics*. Oxford University Press.

Finally, as we discuss morality and ethics, we cannot turn a blind eye to the **abuse of power** in healthcare.[39,40] (In the next category, we quote **Poirier**, who explains how this risk emerges.) The darkest moment in medicine was undoubtedly the role of physicians in the Holocaust. Several scholars, including Reis, propose contemplating the dark and enlightened sides of medicine expressed during these horrible times as a powerful pedagogy for building conscience and morality. How can we immunize ourselves from the inherent risk of abuse of power in medicine? One approach is to foster the moral courage of learners and support speaking up to power when faced with an error or a superior's questionable decision.[41,42,43]

Lesser degrees of abuse and discrimination within the profession also persist. While Kohlberg's theory of moral development was challenged as lacking in feminine care orientation, it also did not incorporate the moral deficiencies arising from racial and gender discrimination (or the additional burdens on women in medicine, especially concerning child and family care) and the widespread phenomenon of microaggressions. Further, it did not address the issue of power in medicine and medical education. These topics are expounded upon in the upcoming categories, particularly in Chapters 7 and 8.

The moral development discourse is ongoing. Recent contributions include Frank's paper and book, in which he describes post-COVID-19 bioethics as a crisis of principles and stories.[44,45] The delicate

39 Reis, S., Wald, H. S., & Weindling, P. (2019). The Holocaust, medicine and becoming a physician: The crucial role of education· *Israel Journal of Health Policy Research*, 8(1), 55. https://doi.org/10.1186/s13584-019-0327-3

40 Reis, S. P., & Wald, H. S. (2015). Contemplating medicine during the Third Reich: Scaffolding professional identity formation for medical students. *Academic Medicine: Journal of the Association of American Medical Colleges*, 90(6), 770–773. https://doi.org/10.1097/ACM.0000000000000716

41 Umoren, R., Kim, S., Gray, M. M., Best, J. A., & Robins, L. (2022). Interprofessional model on speaking up behaviour in healthcare professionals: A qualitative study. *BMJ Leader*, 6(1), 15–19. https://doi.org/10.1136/leader-2020-000407

42 Ellaway, R. H., & Wyatt, T. R. (2021). What role should resistance play in training health professionals? *Academic Medicine: Journal of the Association of American Medical Colleges*, 96(11), 1524–1528. https://doi.org/10.1097/ACM.0000000000004225

43 Bleakley, A. (2020). *Medical education, politics and social justice: The contradiction cure*. Routledge. https://doi.org/10.4324/9781003099093

44 Frank, A. W., & Solbraekke, K. N. (2023). Becoming a cancer survivor: An experiment in dialogical health research. *Health*, 27(1), 78–93. https://doi.org/10.1177/13634593211005178

45 Frank, A. W. (2022). *King Lear: Shakespeare's dark consolations*. Oxford University Press.

TABLE 4.1 Rhodes's Duties of Medical Ethics

1. Seek trust and be deserving of it.
2. Use medical knowledge, skill, powers, privileges, and immunities to promote the interests of patients and society.
3. Develop and maintain professional competence.
4. Provide care based on need.
5. Be mindful in responding to medical needs.
6. Base clinical decisions on scientific evidence.
7. Maintain nonjudgmental regard toward patients.
8. Maintain nonsexual regard toward patients.
9. Maintain the confidentiality of patient information.
10. Respect the autonomy of patients.
11. Assess patients' decisional capacity.
12. Be truthful in your reports.
13. Be responsive to requests from peers.
14. Communicate effectively.
15. Police the profession.
16. Ensure justice in the allocation of medical resources.

Source: Rhodes (2020).

balance between the two was fundamentally disturbed by the pandemic. Principles became politicized, and stories became mediated by group affiliations, consequently preventing dialogue and fueling resistance—often violent—to public health measures such as vaccines and protective gear. Frank predicts the crisis will worsen until bioethics is reinvented. **Rhodes** proposes a new theory of ethics and professionalism.[46] She drafts a list of duties and virtues better aligned with practitioners' moral needs in clinical reality (Table 4.1). Further, she suggests using four virtues—**honesty, diligence, curiosity, and compassion**—as admissions criteria and subsequently reinforcing these in students by facilitating their acquisition of the 16 duties.

From Kalet's opening story to the discussions throughout this chapter, healthcare does not occur in a vacuum and is always molded and challenged by powerful structural forces. Wars are one example, state ideologies and dictates are another; so are economic and social upheavals, as well as pandemics. While we wish for health practitioners to possess moral agency and the courage and ability to speak up when necessary, and aim to facilitate these traits in their formation, we must recognize that learners and practitioners may find themselves in circumstances where they must compromise and sometimes forsake values in order to survive. The experience of the physician in these realities deserves better

---

46 Rhodes, R. (2020). *The trusted doctor: Medical ethics and professionalism.* Oxford University Press.

description, and inquiry into how moral development and behavior, empathy, compassion, clinical judgment, professional identity, professional development, and practice are influenced becomes a priority.

Summary

This category is the fourth to describe a developmental stage model, this time concerning physician moral development. The opening story is a reminder of the current distressing cataclysms of war, where ethical transgressions abound and humanitarian as well as healthcare crises also challenge medicine and health professionals. This category traces the evolution of the construct of physician moral development up to its current complex understanding. At present, it incorporates the ethics of care into principled ethics and examines the gap between the moral ideal and moral reality, as well as the view of moral distress and injury as foundational. This construct also highlights the daunting propensity to abuse power, which challenges physicians throughout their careers, especially when in dire straits such as war and/or when faced with an overwhelming refugee crisis. Again, scholars point out that most physicians do not reach their potential in moral and character development. Will medicine take on the plea to make prevention and care of mass atrocities integral to both identity and competence? Will Frank's forecast of the need to reinvent bioethics materialize (see Chapter 10)? Can these issues be integrated into the former and subsequent categories?

REFERENCES

Baldwin, D. C., Jr, Daugherty, S., & Self, D. J. (1991). Changes in moral reasoning during medical school. *Academic Medicine: Journal of the Association of American Medical Colleges, 66*(Suppl 9), S1, 1–3.

Beauchamp, T. L., & Childress, J. F. (2001). *Principles of biomedical ethics.* Oxford University Press.

Bebeau, M. J. (2009). Enhancing professionalism using ethics education as part of a dental licensure board's disciplinary action. Part 2. Evidence of the process. *Journal of the American College of Dentists, 76*(3), 32–45.

Bebeau, M. J., & Thoma, S. J. (1999). "Intermediate" concepts and the connection to moral education. *Educational Psychology Review, 11*(4), 343–360. https://psycnet.apa.org/doi/10.1023/A:1022057316180

Bebeau, M. J. (2002). The defining issues test and the four-component model: Contributions to professional education. *Journal of Moral Education, 31*(3), 271–295. https://doi.org/10.1080/0305724022000008115

Bebeau, M. J. (2006). Evidence based character development. In N. P. Kenny & W. Shelton (Eds.), Lost virtue: Professional character development in medical education. *Advances in Bioethics, 10,* 47–86. https://doi.org/10.1016/S1479-3709(06)10004-7

Bebeau, M. J. (2009). Enhancing professionalism using ethics education as part of a dental licensure board's disciplinary action. Part 1. An evidence-based process. *Journal of the American College of Dentists*, 76(2), 38–50.

Bebeau, M. J., & Monson, V. E. (2012). Professional identity formation and transformation across the life span. In A. Mc Kee & M. Eraut (Eds.), *Learning trajectories, innovation and identity for professional development* (pp. 135–162). Springer. https://doi.org/10.1007/978-94-007-1724-4_7

Bleakley, A. (2020). *Medical education, politics and social justice: The contradiction cure*. Routledge. https://doi.org/10.4324/9781003099093

Brooks, L., & Bell, D. (2017). Teaching, learning and assessment of medical ethics at the UK medical schools. *Journal of Medical Ethics*, 43(9), 606–612. https://doi.org/10.1136/medethics-2015-103189

Bryan, C. S., & Babelay, A. M. (2009). Building character: A model for reflective practice. *Academic Medicine: Journal of the Association of American Medical Colleges*, 84(9), 1283–1288. https://doi.org/10.1097/ACM.0b013e3181b6a79c

Czech, H., Hildebrandt, S., Reis, S. P., Chelouche, T., Fox, M., González-López, E., Lepicard, E., Ley, A., Offer, M., Ohry, A., Rotzoll, M., Sachse, C., Siegel, S. J., Šimůnek, M., Teicher, A., Uzarczyk, K., von Villiez, A., Wald, H. S., Wynia, M. K., & Roelcke, V. (2023). The Lancet Commission on medicine, Nazism, and the Holocaust: Historical evidence, implications for today, teaching for tomorrow. *Lancet*, 402(10415), 1867–1940. https://doi.org/10.1016/S0140-6736(23)01845-7

Ellaway, R. H., & Wyatt, T. R. (2021). What role should resistance play in training health professionals? *Academic Medicine: Journal of the Association of American Medical Colleges*, 96(11), 1524–1528. https://doi.org/10.1097/ACM.0000000000004225

Fatima, S. (2016). Can doctors maintain good character? An examination of physician lives. *Journal of Medical Humanities*, 37(4), 419–433. https://doi.org/10.1007/s10912-016-9385-5

Ford, E. W. (2019). Stress, burnout, and moral injury: The state of the healthcare workforce. *Journal of Healthcare Management/American College of Healthcare Executives*, 64(3), 125–127. https://doi.org/10.1097/JHM-D-19-00058

Frank, A. W. (2022). *King Lear: Shakespeare's dark consolations*. Oxford University Press.

Frank, A. W., & Solbraekke, K. N. (2023). Becoming a cancer survivor: An experiment in dialogical health research. *Health*, 27(1), 78–93. https://doi.org/10.1177/13634593211005178

Gilligan, C. (1982). *In a different voice: Psychological theory and women's development*. Harvard University Press.

Hawking, M., Curlin, F. A., & Yoon, J. D. (2017). Courage and compassion: Virtues in caring for so-called "difficult" patients. *JAMA Ethics* 19(4), 357–363. https://doi.org/10.1001/journalofethics.2017.19.4.medu2-1704

Jakubowski, H., Xie, J., Kumar Mitra, A., Ghooi, R., Hosseinkhani, S., Alipour, M., Hajipour, B., & Obiero, G. (2017). The global ethics corner: Foundations, beliefs, and the teaching of biomedical and scientific ethics around the world. *Biochemistry and Molecular Biology Education: A Bimonthly Publication of the International Union of Biochemistry and Molecular Biology*, 45(5), 385–395. https://doi.org/10.1002/bmb.21059

Kalet, A. (2022, April 22). What is going on in Ukraine will change us forever. *Transformational Times: Newsletter of the Robert D. and Patricia E. Kern Institute for the Transformation of Medical Education*.

Kim, D. T., Applewhite, M. K., & Shelton, W. (2023). Professional identity formation in medical education: Some virtue-based insights. *Teaching and Learning in Medicine*, 1–11. Advance online publication. https://doi.org/10.1080/10401334.2023.2209067

Kleinman, A. (2013). From illness as culture to caregiving as moral experience. *New England Journal of Medicine*, *368*(15), 1376–1377. https://doi.org/10.1056/NEJMp1300678

Kleinman, A. (2006). *What really matters: Living a moral life amidst uncertainty and danger* (1st ed.). Oxford University Press.

Kleinman, A. (2014). How we endure. *Lancet*, *383*(9912), 119–120. https://doi.org/10.1016/s0140-6736(14)60012-x

Kleinman, A. (2016). Caring for memories. *Lancet*, *387*(10038), 2596–2597. https://doi.org/10.1016/s0140-6736(16)30853-4

Kleinman, A. (2019). *The soul of care: The moral education of a husband and doctor.* Viking.

Kotzee, B., & Ignatowicz, A. (2016). Measuring 'virtue' in medicine. *Medicine, Health Care, and Philosophy*, *19*(2), 149–161. https://doi.org/10.1007/s11019-015-9653-6

Lessing, J. N., Bryan, S., Johnson, C., Keating, J., & Guerrasio, J. (2019). Junior doctor remediation: An international reflection. *Medical Journal of Australia*, *211*(11), 507–508.e1. https://doi.org/10.5694/mja2.50422

Molinaro, M. L., Shen, K., Agarwal, G., Inglis, G., & Vanstone, M. (2023). Family physicians' moral distress when caring for patients experiencing social inequities: A critical narrative inquiry in primary care. *British Journal of General Practice: The Journal of the Royal College of General Practitioners*, *74*(738), e41–e48. https://doi.org/10.3399/BJGP.2023.0193

Monson, V., Bebeau, M. J., Faber-Langendoen, K., & Kalet, A. (2023). Professionalism lapses as professional identity formation challenges. In A. Kalet & C. L. Chou (Eds.), *Remediation in medical education* (pp. 147–161). Springer. https://doi.org/10.1007/978-3-031-32404-8

Patenaude, J., Niyonsenga, T., & Fafard, D. (2003). Changes in the components of moral reasoning during students' medical education: A pilot study. *Medical Education*, *37*(9), 822–829. https://doi.org/10.1046/j.1365-2923.2003.01593.x

Regehr, G. (2006). The persistent myth of stability. On the chronic underestimation of the role of context in behavior. *Journal of General Internal Medicine*, *21*(5), 544–545. https://doi.org/10.1111/j.1525-1497.2006.00447.x

Reis, S. P., & Wald, H. S. (2015). Contemplating medicine during the Third Reich: Scaffolding professional identity formation for medical students. *Academic Medicine: Journal of the Association of American Medical Colleges*, *90*(6), 770–773. https://doi.org/10.1097/ACM.0000000000000716

Reis, S. P., & Wald, H. S. (2024). The Hamas massacre of Oct 7, 2023, and its aftermath, medical crimes, and the Lancet Commission report on medicine, Nazism, and the Holocaust. *Israel Journal of Health Policy Research*, *13*(1), 19. https://doi.org/10.1186/s13584-024-00608-w

Reis, S. P., Wald, H. S., & Weindling, P. (2019). The Holocaust, medicine and becoming a physician: The crucial role of education. *Israel Journal of Health Policy Research*, *8*(1), 55. https://doi.org/10.1186/s13584-019-0327-3

Rest, J. R. (1993). Research on moral judgment in college students. In A. Garrod (Ed.), *Approaches to moral development: New research and emerging themes* (pp. 201–213). Teachers College Press.

Rest, J. R., Thoma, S. J., & Edwards, L. (1997). Designing and validating a measure of moral judgment: Stage preference and stage consistency approaches. *Journal of Educational Psychology*, *89*(1), 5–28. https://doi.org/10.1037/0022-0663.89.1.5

Rest, J., Narvaez, D., Bebeau, M., & Thoma, S. (1999). A neo-Kohlbergian approach: The DIT and schema theory. *Educational Psychology Review*, *11*(4), 291–324. https://doi.org/10.1023/A:1022053215271

Rhodes, R. (2020). *The trusted doctor: Medical ethics and professionalism.* Oxford University Press.

Self, D. J., Baldwin, D. C., Jr, & Wolinsky, F. D. (1992). Evaluation of teaching medical ethics by an assessment of moral reasoning. *Medical Education*, 26(3), 178–184. https://doi.org/10.1111/j.1365-2923.1992.tb00151.x

Skelton, J. R., Wiskin, C. M., & Ward, J. D. T. (2019). Understanding professional development: Case studies of remedial support. *Medical Teacher*, 41(12), 1372–1379. https://doi.org/10.1080/0142159X.2019.1638896

Thaxton, R. E., Jones, W. S., Hafferty, F. W., April, C. W., & April, M. D. (2018). Self vs. other focus: Predicting professionalism remediation of emergency medicine residents. *Western Journal of Emergency Medicine*, 19(1), 35–40. https://doi.org/10.5811/westjem.2017.11.35242

Umoren, R., Kim, S., Gray, M. M., Best, J. A., & Robins, L. (2022). Interprofessional model on speaking up behaviour in healthcare professionals: A qualitative study. *BMJ Leader*, 6(1), 15–19. https://doi.org/10.1136/leader-2020-000407

Waldman, R. A., Waldman, S. D., & Carter, B. S. (2019). When I say... moral distress as a teaching point. *Medical Education*, 53(5), 430–431. https://doi.org/10.1111/medu.13769

Walker, L. J. (2002). The model and the measure: An appraisal of the Minnesota approach to moral development. *Journal of Moral Education*, 31(3), 353–367. https://doi.org/10.1080/0305724022000008160

CHAPTER 5

Narrative, storytelling, and reflection

The handling of emotions

....

The "difficult" patient who taught me radical love

It is July 4, 1984, I am on call for the first time. My resident is terse on the phone. "Sandra's in the ER. She's an emancipated minor in DKA with a blood pH of 6.90! Get down there STAT and escort her to the ICU." He races through her other labs. I grab my things and hustle down to the emergency room, preparing to meet my very first patient. She sounds sick.

On the way, I run my mental checklist of everything I know about DKA, diabetic ketoacidosis. She will need intravenous fluids, insulin, potassium replacement, and oxygen, I think. Given her labs, I expect she will be comatose and on a ventilator. I wonder what my resident meant when he said she is an "emancipated minor." I'll figure it out.

Clutching my new clipboard to my chest, I walk tentatively into the emergency room where my eyes are drawn to a bizarre scene. A tiny barefoot girl with a blonde pixie haircut and white, nearly translucent skin is screaming at two psychiatry residents and two burly, armed hospital police officers. She effectively holds them at bay using an IV pole like a lance. Her hospital gown hangs loosely and bright red blood drips from her wrist where she has partially removed her arterial line. As I watch, she unleashes an impressive, incongruent stream of obscenities. I am spellbound as the four men warily circle the child.

A firm hand on my shoulder breaks the spell. I look up to see Dr. Lewis Goldfrank, one of the ER attendings. He is one of the founders of the specialty of Emergency Medicine and I worked with him last summer as a visiting student. He is very tall, slim, and looks not unlike Abraham Lincoln. "Sandra will be yours, Adina," he says gently.

DOI: 10.1201/9781003507529-6

Before I can register his comment, Pixie Cut slams down the IV pole and streaks past me and into a bathroom. The door slams and the lock clicks. Goldfrank smiles and shrugs. "You need to get her out of there before she loses consciousness, and we have to call Engineering to take down the door." He seems unperturbed.

Deeply grateful for his support, I crouch down outside the bathroom. I talk to Sandra through the keyhole. Twenty minutes later she acquiesces and opens the door, probably because she is getting sicker and can't keep up the fight.

I lead her back to bed, trying to ignore her attempts to spit on me. My resident and I place new IVs and restart her lifesaving treatments. As 16-year-olds are wont to do, Sandra quickly improves. She nods off.

While she sleeps, I head down to Medical Records. Her paper chart is surprisingly sparse. The first page, from when she was six years old, is from an ER visit when she was brought in with multiple contusions and broken bones. That admission led to a long hospitalization which ended when Child Protective Services removed her from her mother's chaotic home and placed her in foster care.

I sag to the ground, overwhelmed with sadness for Sandra as a little girl. I sob (it has been a long and exhausting day). I realize what "emancipated" *really* means for her: as a homeless, chronically ill adolescent who was severely abused as a child, she can be admitted to the hospital without notifying a parent or guardian. As an emancipated minor, though, she can also refuse care, which she routinely does.

I discover she has been admitted to hospitals all over New York City. There are notes about her marginal living arrangements and claims of possible drug use. At some point, someone figures out that she is diabetic and should be on insulin. She never stays in the hospital long enough to learn diabetes management, work with social services, or receive psychiatric care. She never follows up. She doesn't have one of the psychiatric diagnoses that allows her to be involuntarily admitted for her own safety, even for a short time. Every discharge summary reflects a sense of resignation.

I close her medical record file and head back up to the ER. For now, she will be my responsibility. In fact, she will be my responsibility intermittently for the next three full years.

About once a month she appears in our ER. Because she has an untreated life-threatening illness, she is always seen. Depending on her mood, she asks the ER team to call me, and whenever she is told that admissions are assigned in a strict rotation and that "Dr. Kalet is not on call today," she begins to scream my name. Before long, and with Dr. Goldfrank's approval, someone finds me to come and see my "special admission."

As soon as she can, she bolts from the hospital against medical advice without her medications or any follow-up arrangements. One time, I talk her into setting up a visit to see me in clinic where we have a nurse practitioner expert in diabetes care, but she never shows. Occasionally, I speak to other physicians who have connected with her, and we try to find some way to "manage her," but she never cooperates.

I try unsuccessfully to avoid Sandra. I am terrified by her self-destructive behavior. I find her draining and disheartening to care for medically.

It is very, very frustrating. As a group, and usually over late-night cups of cold coffee, my residency colleagues and I debate whether she "deserves" the expensive, all but futile medical management she makes so difficult to provide. Why should we care for or about her? I am no saint, and when I hear that she is back in the ER demanding to "see Dr. Kalet," I want to turn and run, wishing to avoid the predictable and exasperating burden she lays on me.

With time, though, things evolve. Over the course of Sandra's many hospitalizations, I sit at her bedside, rather than in the doctor's station, to chart her glucose, potassium, blood pH, oxygen levels, and kidney and liver functions. I become comfortable managing diabetic ketoacidosis and discover its fascinating physiology. When she becomes enraged and uncooperative, the nurses call and, sometimes, I am able to convince her to undergo diagnostic testing or treatment for her infections.

We develop a tentative connection. Once my empathy is activated by her origin story, I feel morally obligated to stay in a relationship with her and to never stop trying to help. What I feel is unconditional, transcendent, and persistent regardless of the circumstances. I can't bring myself to *not* feel love for this difficult child. In fact, what I feel for Sandra—and what Dr. Goldfrank insists I learn to feel for Sandra—is "radical love."

In retrospect, I realize now that I *loved* Sandra, despite not *liking* her.

Ancient Greek philosophers described several different kinds of "love." *Agape*, or what they called "love of mankind," is essential to our humanity despite not always being particularly pleasurable. It does not always easily align with the analytical reasoning needed to be a technically competent physician.

Theologians, philosophers, and poets throughout the ages, and modern "social justice warriors" such as Martin Luther King, Jr., considered this kind of love radical and powerful. As Dr. King said, "It's difficult to like some people. But *love* is greater than *like*. Love is understanding and creative, redemptive good will." The late bell hooks added that Dr. King "believed that love is 'ultimately the only answer' to the problems facing this nation and the entire planet." I knew none of that at the time when I was caring for Sandra, but I can see now how it affected me and how I experienced my relationship with her.

One day, after we have known each other for a couple of years, her diabetes lands her back in the hospital. Sensing an opening, I walk in with a pad and pen, intent on finally teaching her about insulin dosing (this was before insulin pumps were available). I sit on her bed and draw pictures. I write out careful instructions. For a long time, she is engaged. Then, because I want to make certain that she is "getting it," I ask her to read the notes back to me. She becomes enraged.

"Get out!" she screams. "I hate you!" I realize too late that she cannot read.

I do not know what to do. I turn my back and walk toward the door.

Suddenly, her lunch tray, including her knives, forks, and all of her food, crashes to the floor behind me. I angrily turn around. "Hey, you could have hurt me!" I yell.

She stares back defiantly. "If I had wanted to hit you, I would have!"
I soften. *Touché!* I think. I guess, in her own way, Sandra loves me, too.[1]

* * *

The opening story of the fifth category is a physician's narrative of tough love within a clinical relationship with a very challenging patient. It relays aspects that are usually foreign to the clinical discourse—feelings, inner conflict, distress—and invites the reader to engage in a parallel inner discourse. In the previous category, difficult patients were qualified as a "moral stress test" for moral development. The story here both illustrates this observation and conveys its lived experience, as narratives should.

STORYTELLING AND NARRATIVE COMPETENCE

By now, narrative medicine (NM), reflective writing, and narrative competence literature are extensive,[2,3,4,5,6,7,8,9,10] promoting "narrative

1 Kalet, A. (2022). The "difficult" patient who taught me radical love. *Transformational Times: Newsletter of the Robert D. and Patricia E. Kern Institute for the Transformation of Medical Education.*

2 Milota, M. M., van Thiel, G. J. M. W., & van Delden, J. J. M. (2019). Narrative medicine as a medical education tool: A systematic review. *Medical Teacher*, 41(7), 802–810. https://doi.org/10.1080/0142159X.2019.1584274

3 Leopold, S. S. (2018). Editorial: What is narrative medicine, and why should we use it in orthopaedic practice? *Clinical Orthopaedics and Related Research*, 476(11), 2105–2107. https://doi.org/10.1097/CORR.0000000000000504

4 Murphy, J. W., Franz, B. A., & Schlaerth, C. (2018). The role of reflection in narrative medicine. *Journal of Medical Education and Curricular Development*, 5. https://doi.org/10.1177/2382120518785301

5 Pulse: Voices from the Heart of Medicine. What is Pulse? https://pulsevoices.org/about/what-is-pulse/

6 Chen, P. J., Huang, C. D., & Yeh, S. J. (2017). Impact of a narrative medicine programme on healthcare providers' empathy scores over time. *BMC Medical Education*, 17(1), 108. https://doi.org/10.1186/s12909-017-0952-x

7 Weiss, T., & Swede, M. J. (2019). Transforming preprofessional health education through relationship-centered care and narrative medicine. *Teaching and Learning in Medicine*, 31(2), 222–233. https://doi.org/10.1080/10401334.2016.1159566

8 Chretien, K. C., Swenson, R., Yoon, B., Julian, R., Keenan, J., Croffoot, J., & Kheirbek, R. (2015). Tell me your story: A pilot narrative medicine curriculum during the medicine clerkship. *Journal of General Internal Medicine*, 30(7), 1025–1028. https://doi.org/10.1007/s11606-015-3211-z

9 Miller, E., Balmer, D., Hermann, N., Graham, G., & Charon, R. (2014). Sounding narrative medicine: Studying students' professional identity development at Columbia University College of Physicians and Surgeons. *Academic Medicine: Journal of the Association of American Medical Colleges*, 89(2), 335–342. https://doi.org/10.1097/ACM.0000000000000098

10 Charon, R. (2007). What to do with stories: The sciences of narrative medicine. *Canadian Family Physician/Medecin de famille canadien*, 53(8), 1265–1267.

competence as a teachable mode of practicing evidence-based medicine with the skills of active listening, close reading and narrative writing." It has also been mentioned in all the former categories.

Avrahami and **Reis** write:

> Physicians have stories that demand to be told. … Not only those of patients but of their lay and professional caretakers as well. … Narrative Medicine, or medicine practiced with narrative skills, considers the stories of patients and their caretakers as integral to the experience of ill health and healing. In Europe, the United States, Canada, and Israel, NM researchers and facilitators have begun to investigate the development of physicians' sensibility to language and promote narrative competence.[11]

In the literature on narrative medicine, a correlation is repeatedly identified between reflective capacity, clinical reasoning, and diagnostic acumen (previously mentioned in Chapter 3). As such, "soft" (we prefer to call them basic, core, or intrinsic) competencies may actually be instrumental as clinical skills and therefore shift from the "nice to have" status to essential and even lifesaving.[12] Reflection is thus a capability that is foundational to clinical reasoning as well as to personal and professional growth, identity formation, and moral development.

The number of memoirs of the journey through medical school and residency—sometimes beyond, with rare accounts of entire lifespans—is growing exponentially.[13] Curiously, this is almost exclusively a North American phenomenon. Furthermore, journals (*NEJM*, *JAMA*, *Annals of Internal Medicine*, *Pulse*, *Lancet*, *BMJ*, and more) are regularly publishing physician narratives which offer "laments" and "awakenings." When analyzed as a dataset, these provide insights concerning what is presently on physicians' minds.[14] In addition to memoirs of the formative years, physician illness narratives recounting experiences of personal

---

11 Avrahami, E., & Reis, S. (2009). Narrative medicine. *Israel Medical Association Journal: IMAJ, 11*(6), 335–338.

12 Lafleur, A., Gagné, M., Paquin, V., & Michaud-Couture, C. (2019). How to convince clinicians that 'soft' skills save lives? Practical tips to use clinical studies to teach physicians' roles. *MedEdPublish, 8*, 119. https://doi.org/10.15694/mep.2019.000119.1

13 Moniz, T., Costella, J., Golafshani, M., Watling, C., & Lingard, L. (2021). Bringing narratives from physicians, patients and caregivers together: A scoping review of published research. *Medical Humanities, 47*(1), 27–37. https://doi.org/10.1136/medhum-2017-011424

14 Schei, E., Fuks, A., & Boudreau, J. D. (2019). Reflection in medical education: Intellectual humility, discovery, and know-how. *Medicine, Health Care, and Philosophy, 22*(2), 167–178. https://doi.org/10.1007/s11019-018-9878-2

ill-health (such as the opening narrative of Chapter 6) are multiplying, thereby sensitizing reader-physicians to their vulnerability and shared humanity.[15] Other narratives are faculty tales, which facilitate both the narrators' personal and professional identity formation[16] and that of the residents they mentor.[17]

Bryant investigates eight novels with medical student protagonists.[18] He writes:

> These heroes have had much in common. They start out poor, handi-capped, virtually if not actually fatherless. Soon, in the laboratories of dreary or ominous institutions, and in the classrooms of inept, insensi-tive teachers; they encounter a stylized Death which goes on to haunt them in the shrouds of personal illness and mortal fears. Paralleling this irony of healers as victims, alienated from life and self, runs the threat of alienation from medicine and idealism. Ultimately they return from their brush with mortality and with professional despair, and succeed in their quest to become physicians, even extraordinary ones, and whole human beings.
>
> (p. 250)

Frank[19] categorizes physician narratives into success, chaos, and quest stories. He also highlights the notion of the wounded healer[20] as an essential element of physician development, self-awareness, and human-ism (see Chapter 6).

This is the second category that acknowledges **race talk and feminist narratives**. In their chapter in *The Principles and Practice of Narrative Medicine* by **Charon** et al., **Spiegel** and **Spencer** write:

15 Bahri, D. (2022). Why stories about illness matter. *Lancet*, 399(10340), 2009–2010. https://doi.org/10.1016/S0140-6736(22)00933-3

16 Mema, B., Helmers, A., Anderson, C., Min, K. K., & Navne, L. E. (2021). Who am I? Narratives as a window to transformative moments in critical care. *PLoS One*, 16(11), e0259976. https://doi.org/10.1371/journal.pone.0259976

17 Khoo, S. M., & Wong, X. L. S. (2022). When faculty tell tales: How faculty members' reflective narratives impact residents' professional identity formation. *Academic Medicine: Journal of the Association of American Medical Colleges*, 97(3), 385–388. https://doi.org/10.1097/ACM.0000000000004256

18 Bryant, D. C. (1996). Telling tales out of school—Portrayals of the medical student experience by physician-novelists. *Journal of Medical Humanities*, 17(4), 237–254. https://doi.org/10.1007/BF02276871

19 Frank, A. W. (2000). The standpoint of storyteller. *Qualitative Health Research* 10(3), 354-365. https://doi.org/10.1177/104973200129118499

20 Frank, A. W. (1995). *The wounded storyteller: Body, illness and ethics*. The University of Chicago Press.

Feminists and race theorists recognize both the pedagogical and *political* value of learning to speak about feelings in the classroom. As Derald Wing Sue describes in *Race Talk and the Conspiracy of Silence*,[21,22] students appreciate instructors who are unafraid to recognize the racial tension that can emerge in class discussion and to name the feelings that can attend it: "The skilled facilitator helps others make sense of these feelings and frees the individual from being controlled by them. As long as feelings remain unnamed and unacknowledged, they represent emotional roadblocks to having a successful dialogue."[23]

(p. 38)

THE INNER LIVES OF STUDENTS AND DOCTORS

In her pioneering work, Poirier analyzes accounts of medical school and residency education experiences in the United States published between 1965 and 2005.[24] In these narratives, she finds evidence of how young women and men come to view themselves, their patients, and the moral nature of their work. Their patterns "soon become predictable. ... Similar dilemmas involving patients, sources of distress or satisfaction, and values by which the writer judges his or her teachers. ... The causes of grief and joy for the authors remain basically unchanged." A special aspect is that of embodiment:

I catalog how the corporeal nature of medical education and practice becomes lodged in the writers' language and metaphors of memory ... how writers document their relationship to their own bodies and the bodies of patients, how the physical work of medical education reveals the vulnerability that is an inherent part of becoming a physician, and how medical students and residents frame their search for professional integrity in opposition to definitions of the physician's body that are generally held by their teachers.

The authors, Poirier notes, "represent medical education as a process that is inherently embodied; these passages lodge specific events of patient care in the physicians' very brains, hands, and feet." This involves "an

---

21 Sue, D. W., & Spanierman, L. (2020). *Microaggressions in everyday life* (2nd ed.). John Wiley & Sons.

22 Sue, D. W. (2016). *Race talk and the conspiracy of silence: Understanding facilitating difficult dialogues on race.* John Wiley & Sons.

23 Charon, R. (2017). *The principles and practice of narrative medicine.* Oxford University Press.

24 Poirier, S. (2009). *Doctors in the making: Memoirs and medical education.* University of Iowa Press.

inescapable distancing of the self from its body and … the very expression of the body's desires, especially concerning vulnerability and mortality."

Dreams are most frequently acknowledged as repositories of memories in these accounts. Nearly every memoir describes one, often recurring dream that "haunts, taunts, or chastises the dreamer" (remember Marcus's study of medical school students' dreams discussed in Chapter 1). Poirier identifies the **performative nature** of being a physician and the multiple vulnerabilities that it evokes (recall Marcus again). One example is the tension, especially in surgery, between self-perception and expectations when learning a procedure. This is another, possibly necessary step whereby the body is dissociated from emotions on the way to gaining technical expertise.

Regarding the propensity to abuse power (also discussed in Chapter 4), Poirier writes of a "thin line between therapy and assault." In addition to **gender and race, sexuality** is a major focus in academic examinations of embodiment: in "instances when the writer's sexuality becomes a conscious part of his or her work … sexuality becomes one of several kinds of experiences that register as a physical threat to the student or resident."

Further, Poirier notices metaphysical debates between **one's self and one's self as physician,** which reveal the complex dynamic of body, culture, and psyche in the shaping of the professional identity: "Nurses' memoirs … trace the trajectory of burnout … a bottomless well of selfless caring often denies the emotional effects of such work on the nurse herself. … [Ascribing] their patients with the potential for physical threat," including infection and physical force, is vulnerability. As are the lack of sleep, exhaustion, and debilitation that beget demoralization, loss of compassion, self-pity, and finally patient blaming. "Paradoxically, fear of personal vulnerability, whether physical or psychological, can lead to abuse of power of which the practitioner is at least temporarily oblivious."

Poirier's powerful analysis highlights how medicine is embodied, how this corporality inevitably anchors the field in the physical and emotional vulnerabilities that all humans share. Thus, her work fosters humility and emotional honesty, in contrast to the dissociation from emotions heralded in the past.[25,26] She views the formation of physicians as a sequence of "very specific moral landmarks … changing conscience and self-confidence," whereby the potential for **loss of perspective and abuse of power** become recognized. Finally, "his own sense of moral

25 Vinson, A. H., & Underman, K. (2020). Clinical empathy as emotional labor in medical work. *Social Science & Medicine, 251,* 112904. https://doi.org/10.1016/j.socscimed.2020.112904

26 Dornan, T., Pearson, E., Carson, P., Helmich, E., & Bundy, C. (2015). Emotions and identity in the figured world of becoming a doctor. *Medical Education, 49*(2), 174–185. https://doi.org/10.1111/medu.12587

vulnerability is a necessary condition for his performance of his profession's knowledge and power." Poirier's work resonates strongly with the previous category, as well as the upcoming one.

Shapiro, another narrative scholar, employs the reflective writing of emerging and established health professionals as her data.[27] She has carefully traced how, even in the present days of humanizing the curriculum, co-creation and perpetuation of "professional alexithymia"[28] (dissociation from emotions) are dominant in the hidden curriculum. She offers a compelling perspective as to why the development of desired professional empathy encounters such barriers and hardly becomes integrated into the evolving professional identities. In a seminal paper, she argues that learners' basic "emotional responses to the universal human vulnerability to illness, disability, decay, and ultimately death that they must confront in the process of rendering patient care" are "complex, and mostly unresolved," and that "in the absence of appropriate discourses about how to emotionally manage distressing aspects of the human condition, it is likely that trainees will resort to coping mechanisms that result in distance and detachment." Such a response is rooted in human nature:

> The impulse to "draw closer," to become engaged and connected with the suffering other, is far from automatic in human nature. In fact, we have an equal, if not stronger, and opposite impulse to draw back, detach, and separate from the contamination of illness.

Shapiro proceeds by expounding on how human identity is constituted as much by "othering" (negative identity: demarcation of the sick, disabled, or dying as other) as it is by positive identity. When coupled with "modernist assumptions about the capacity to protect, control, and restore [that] run deep," this intra-subjective process "can create barriers to empathic relationships." Shapiro identifies:

> [There is a] need for an epistemological paradigm that helps trainees develop a tolerance for imperfection in self and others; and acceptance of shared emotional vulnerability and suffering while simultaneously honoring the existence of difference. Reducing the sense of anxiety and

---

27 Shapiro, J. (2008). Walking a mile in their patients' shoes: Empathy and othering in medical students' education. *Philosophy, Ethics, and Humanities in Medicine: PEHM*, 3(10). https://doi.org/10.1186/1747-5341-3-10

28 Shapiro, J. (2011). Perspective: Does medical education promote professional alexithymia? A call for attending to the emotions of patients and self in medical training. *Academic Medicine: Journal of the Association of American Medical Colleges*, 86(3), 326–332. https://doi.org/10.1097/ACM.0b013e3182088833

threat that are now reinforced by the dominant medical discourse in the presence of illness will enable trainees to learn to emotionally contain the suffering of their patients and themselves, thus providing a psychologically sound foundation for the development of true empathy.

Finally, Shapiro suggests an **ethos of imperfection** as a framework that should replace the ones identified as presently prevalent, providing a detailed proposal for operationalizing this framework in medical education.

REFLECTIVE PRACTICE

The review of the literature presented in this category validates Schön, who was the first to describe reflective practice.[29,30] An allusion to the epistemology (conceptual clarity) of reflective practice seems helpful. Kinsella summarized the epistemological underpinnings of reflective practice as follows: "(1) A broad critique of technical rationality; (2) professional practice knowledge as artistry; (3) constructivist assumptions in the theory; (4) the significance of tacit knowledge for professional practice knowledge; and (5) overcoming mind body dualism to recognize the knowledge revealed in intelligent action."[31]

Recently, reports on the use of reflective writing to study and measure professional identity formation (PIF) abound.[32,33,34,35,36] More on this in Chapter 9.

29 Schon, D. A. (1984). *The reflective practitioner: How professionals think in action.* Basic Books.
30 Schon, D. A. (1987). *Educating the reflective practitioner: Toward a new design for teaching and learning in the professions.* Jossey-Bass.
31 Kinsella, E. A. (2010). Professional knowledge and the epistemology of reflective practice. *Nursing Philosophy: An International Journal for Healthcare Professionals, 11*(1), 3–14. https://doi.org/10.1111/j.1466-769X.2009.00428.x
32 Lim, J. Y., Ong, S. Y. K., Ng, C. Y. H., Chan, K. L. E., Wu, S. Y. E. A., So, W. Z., Tey, G. J. C., Lam, Y. X., Gao, N. L. X., Lim, Y. X., Tay, R. Y. K., Leong, I. T. Y., Rahman, N. D. A., Chiam, M., Lim, C., Phua, G. L. G., Murugam, V., Ong, E. K., & Krishna, L. K. R. (2023). A systematic scoping review of reflective writing in medical education. *BMC Medical Education, 23*(1), 12. https://doi.org/10.1186/s12909-022-03924-4
33 Makarem, N. N., Rahme, D. V., Brome, D., & Saab, B. R. (2023). Grading reflective essays: The construct validity and reliability of a newly developed Tool- GRE-9. *BMC Medical Education, 23*(1), 870. https://doi.org/10.1186/s12909-023-04845-6
34 Kuhn, J., Mamede, S., van den Berg, P., Zwaan, L., Elshout, G., Bindels, P., & van Gog, T. (2024). Teaching medical students to apply deliberate reflection. *Medical Teacher, 46*(1), 65–72. https://doi.org/10.1080/0142159X.2023.2229504
35 Schaepkens, S. P. C., de la Croix, A., & Veen, M. (2024). 'Oh yes, that is also reflection'—Using discursive psychology to describe how GP registrars construct reflection. *Medical Education, 58*(3), 318–326. https://doi.org/10.1111/medu.15183
36 Talib, M. A., Greene, R. E., & Winkel, A. F. (2024). A narrative analysis of clerkship reflections: Medical student identity development in a changing world. *Clinical Teacher, 21*(1), e13652. https://doi.org/10.1111/tct.13652

Summary

The themes of this narrative category echo those of former, and upcoming, categories. The chapter's opening story, about a transformative clinical experience that engenders radical love in the narrator, is a fine example—alongside the other opening stories in this book—of how accounts of lived experience engage and command deep listening and reflection. The importance of emotions is highlighted, and narrative writing is presented as a practical tool to make room for processing them. Additionally, narratives can help learners and practitioners to process complex experiences, distress, and conflicts, thereby supporting their wellbeing and development. Delving deeper, embodiment, vulnerability, dreams, and empathy are reiterated, and new constructs emerge, such as emotional honesty and an ethos of imperfection, pointing to conditions under which transformation can occur. Further, the narrative nature of clinical reasoning serves as an interface between the expertise category (Chapter 3) and the present narrative one: clinical reasoning draws on reflection, and reflective capacity correlates with diagnostic ability. This category validates narrative medicine and reflective practice as a competence that supports the evolving physician in reaching her full potential above and beyond knowledge, skills, and clinical experience. It also acknowledges in no uncertain terms the impact of components that are relatively absent in the former categories: woundedness, sexuality, race, and gender. In essence, narrative and reflection span all categories and demonstrate that—whatever the lens used—lived experience, self-awareness, and integration of heart and mind are present in the physician life cycle, informing processes and decision-making (ontology before epistemology). They facilitate professional identity formation, clinical performance, wellbeing, and the processing of complex experiences and emotions, as well as support growth from informative to formative and transformative learning. It behooves medical education to integrate them into curricula, pedagogies, and assessment.

REFERENCES

Avrahami, E., & Reis, S. P. (2009). Narrative medicine. *Israel Medical Association Journal: IMAJ*, *11*(6), 335–338.

Bahri, D. (2022). Why stories about illness matter. *Lancet*, *399*(10340), 2009–2010. https://doi.org/10.1016/S0140-6736(22)00933-3

Bryant, D. C. (1996). Telling tales out of school—Portrayals of the medical student experience by physician-novelists. *Journal of Medical Humanities*, *17*(4), 237–254. https://doi.org/10.1007/BF02276871

Charon, R. (2007). What to do with stories: The sciences of narrative medicine. *Canadian Family Physician/Medecin de famille canadien*, *53*(8), 1265–1267.

Charon, R. (2017). *The principles and practice of narrative medicine.* Oxford University Press.

Chen, P. J., Huang, C. D., & Yeh, S. J. (2017). Impact of a narrative medicine programme on healthcare providers' empathy scores over time. *BMC Medical Education, 17*(1), 108. https://doi.org/10.1186/s12909-017-0952-x

Chretien, K. C., Swenson, R., Yoon, B., Julian, R., Keenan, J., Croffoot, J., & Kheirbek, R. (2015). Tell me your story: A pilot narrative medicine curriculum during the medicine clerkship. *Journal of General Internal Medicine, 30*(7), 1025–1028. https://doi.org/10.1007/s11606-015-3211-z

Dornan, T., Pearson, E., Carson, P., Helmich, E., & Bundy, C. (2015). Emotions and identity in the figured world of becoming a doctor. *Medical Education, 49*(2), 174–185. https://doi.org/10.1111/medu.12587

Frank, A. W. (1995). *The wounded storyteller: Body, illness and ethics.* The University of Chicago Press.

Frank, A. W. (2000). Doctors' stories. *Medical Humanities, 14*(2), 72–74.

Kalet, A. (2022). The "difficult" patient who taught me radical love. *Transformational Times: Newsletter of the Robert D. and Patricia E. Kern Institute for the Transformation of Medical Education.*

Khoo, S. M., & Wong, X. L. S. (2022). When faculty tell tales: How faculty members' reflective narratives impact residents' professional identity formation. *Academic Medicine: Journal of the Association of American Medical Colleges, 97*(3), 385–388. https://doi.org/10.1097/ACM.0000000000004256

Kinsella, E. A. (2010). Professional knowledge and the epistemology of reflective practice. *Nursing Philosophy: An International Journal for Healthcare Professionals, 11*(1), 3–14. https://doi.org/10.1111/j.1466-769X.2009.00428.x

Kuhn, J., Mamede, S., van den Berg, P., Zwaan, L., Elshout, G., Bindels, P., & van Gog, T. (2024). Teaching medical students to apply deliberate reflection. *Medical Teacher, 46*(1), 65–72. https://doi.org/10.1080/0142159X.2023.2229504

Lafleur, A., Gagné, M., Paquin, V., & Michaud-Couture, C. (2019). How to convince clinicians that 'soft' skills save lives? Practical tips to use clinical studies to teach physicians' roles. *MedEdPublish, 8,* 119. https://doi.org/10.15694/mep.2019 .000119.1

Leopold, S. S. (2018). Editorial: What is narrative medicine, and why should we use it in orthopaedic practice? *Clinical Orthopaedics and Related Research, 476*(11), 2105–2107. https://doi.org/10.1097/CORR.0000000000000504

Lim, J. Y., Ong, S. Y. K., Ng, C. Y. H., Chan, K. L. E., Wu, S. Y. E. A., So, W. Z., Tey, G. J. C., Lam, Y. X., Gao, N. L. X., Lim, Y. X., Tay, R. Y. K., Leong, I. T. Y., Rahman, N. D. A., Chiam, M., Lim, C., Phua, G. L. G., Murugam, V., Ong, E. K., & Krishna, L. K. R. (2023). A systematic scoping review of reflective writing in medical education. *BMC Medical Education, 23*(1), 12. https://doi.org/10.1186/ s12909-022-03924-4

Makarem, N. N., Rahme, D. V., Brome, D., & Saab, B. R. (2023). Grading reflective essays: The construct validity and reliability of a newly developed Tool- GRE-9. *BMC Medical Education, 23*(1), 870. https://doi.org/10.1186/s12909-023-04845-6

Mema, B., Helmers, A., Anderson, C., Min, K. K., & Navne, L. E. (2021). Who am I? Narratives as a window to transformative moments in critical care. *PLoS One, 16*(11), e0259976. https://doi.org/10.1371/journal.pone.0259976

Miller, E., Balmer, D., Hermann, N., Graham, G., & Charon, R. (2014). Sounding narrative medicine: Studying students' professional identity development at Columbia University College of Physicians and Surgeons. *Academic Medicine: Journal of the Association of American Medical Colleges, 89*(2), 335–342. https:// doi.org/10.1097/ACM.0000000000000098

Milota, M. M., van Thiel, G. J. M. W., & van Delden, J. J. M. (2019). Narrative medicine as a medical education tool: A systematic review. *Medical Teacher*, 41(7), 802–810. https://doi.org/10.1080/0142159X.2019.1584274

Moniz, T., Costella, J., Golafshani, M., Watling, C., & Lingard, L. (2021). Bringing narratives from physicians, patients and caregivers together: A scoping review of published research. *Medical Humanities*, 47(1), 27–37. https://doi.org/10.1136/medhum-2017-011424

Murphy, J. W., Franz, B. A., & Schlaerth, C. (2018). The role of reflection in narrative medicine. *Journal of Medical Education and Curricular Development*, 5. https://doi.org/10.1177/2382120518785301

Poirier, S. (2009). *Doctors in the making: Memoirs and medical education*. University of Iowa Press.

Pulse: Voices from the Heart of Medicine. What is Pulse? https://pulsevoices.org/about/what-is-pulse/

Schaepkens, S. P. C., de la Croix, A., & Veen, M. (2024). 'Oh yes, that is also reflection'— Using discursive psychology to describe how GP registrars construct reflection. *Medical Education*, 58(3), 318–326. https://doi.org/10.1111/medu.15183

Schei, E., Fuks, A., & Boudreau, J. D. (2019). Reflection in medical education: Intellectual humility, discovery, and know-how. *Medicine, Health Care, and Philosophy*, 22(2), 167–178. https://doi.org/10.1007/s11019-018-9878-2

Schon, D. A. (1984). *The reflective practitioner: How professionals think in action*. Basic Books.

Schon, D. A. (1987). *Educating the reflective practitioner: Toward a new design for teaching and learning in the professions*. Jossey-Bass.

Shapiro, J. (2008). Walking a mile in their patients' shoes: Empathy and othering in medical students' education. *Philosophy, Ethics, and Humanities in Medicine: PEHM*, 3(10). https://doi.org/10.1186/1747-5341-3-10

Shapiro, J. (2011). Perspective: Does medical education promote professional alexithymia? A call for attending to the emotions of patients and self in medical training. *Academic Medicine: Journal of the Association of American Medical Colleges*, 86(3), 326–332. https://doi.org/10.1097/ACM.0b013e3182088833

Sue, D. W. (2016). *Race talk and the conspiracy of silence: Understanding facilitating difficult dialogues on race*. John Wiley & Sons.

Sue, D. W., & Spanierman, L. (2020). *Microaggressions in everyday life* (2nd ed.). John Wiley & Sons.

Talib, M. A., Greene, R. E., & Winkel, A. F. (2024). A narrative analysis of clerkship reflections: Medical student identity development in a changing world. *Clinical Teacher*, 21(1), e13652. https://doi.org/10.1111/tct.13652

Vinson, A. H., & Underman, K. (2020). Clinical empathy as emotional labor in medical work. *Social Science & Medicine*, 251, 112904. https://doi.org/10.1016/j.socscimed.2020.112904

Weiss, T., & Swede, M. J. (2019). Transforming preprofessional health education through relationship-centered care and narrative medicine. *Teaching and Learning in Medicine*, 31(2), 222–233. https://doi.org/10.1080/10401334.2016.1159566

CHAPTER 6

Developmental issues, remediation, and the wounded healer

....

Heart attack: A doctor's experience

One in the morning and all is not well! I awaken with burning pain across the front of my chest. My initial reaction is fear: "I wonder if this is my heart."

I can't stand the fear and immediately decide it must be heartburn and go downstairs for an antacid. It doesn't help, and I become fearful again. Then I vomit and convince myself it must be a stomach problem. But the pain gets worse. Finally, I can't bear the pain any longer and ask my wife to call for an ambulance. I decide it is probably a heart attack and take an aspirin. The ambulance arrives in five minutes. The attendants start an IV, give me nitroglycerine, and take me directly to the hospital where I work.

It feels odd to be on the stretcher receiving care rather than providing care. The fear is gone—partly because the pain is so bad that all I can think about is getting relief, and partly because I feel I am in good hands. I see a familiar face, the chief of the ER, looking on, and feel safe. One of the team members does an ECG, and the resident holds it up in front of me where I can easily see the telltale ST elevation indicating an acute MI. They start a nitro drip and administer tPA.

DOI: 10.1201/9781003507529-7

I don't remember anyone discussing my diagnosis or treatment in the ER. It could well have happened, but the experience was such a blur I blotted out much of it. If I gave consent, it was not very informed. But I am not sure I would have wanted to hear about the risk of stroke or death at that time. Finally, the tPA does its job and "busts the clot," my chest pain dissolves, and I go to sleep.

The next day, I meet my cardiologist, hear about my heart attack, and learn that I also have diabetes. I am so glad to be pain-free and alive that I am at peace with this news. I am initially treated with insulin four times a day, as well as with beta-blockers, ramipril, and aspirin to protect my heart, Pravachol to lower my cholesterol, and injections of low molecular weight heparin to prevent a new clot from forming. Again, there is very little discussion of the pros and cons of any of this treatment although I know from professional experience that this is standard therapy.

Later, the doctors decide it is time to switch to oral drugs for my diabetes and tell me they will start glyburide. When I suggest I would prefer metformin, they are hesitant but agree. The next day, my gout flares up, and I ask for NSAIDs. The medication immediately arrives. I am impressed with the rapid response and surprised that there is no discussion.

On the day before discharge, my cardiologist discusses the pros and cons of taking warfarin for a few months and asks if I have any questions or alternative suggestions for therapy. This is the first time anyone has opened up the options, and I am not ready. Although he is sitting down and appears unrushed, I know how busy he is and am hesitant to start a long discussion of the pros and cons of all the different drugs I am on. Despite my professional education and my knowledge of evidence-based medicine, I am intimidated by my vulnerability and don't want to impose on my physician. I want to be a "good" patient.

In reflecting on this experience, I am struck by how vulnerable I felt. Although I spoke up about the treatment of my diabetes and gout (they didn't seem to know how to treat these conditions in the coronary unit), I felt very reluctant to question the treatment of my heart. As an advocate for patient-centered care, I realized how hard it is for patients to have a voice in decisions even when physicians are friendly and invite dialogue. Perhaps doctors need to take the time over several visits to present treatment options and to explicitly address patient reluctance to question authority. As I return to practice, I understand more fully the tremendous power differential between patients and doctors, and use my experience to try to bridge that gap and encourage my patients to give voice to their ideas and concerns.[1]

* * *

1   W. W. Weston. Unpublished personal narrative.

THE WOUNDED HEALER

Health professional woundedness may result, as in the opening narrative of this chapter, from a health problem. Physicians experience illness like all humans. However, their share of mental illness, addiction, and suicide is greater than that of the general population, and their coping, as well as how they are both cared for and viewed by their colleagues, is distinct. **Wilson** et al.[2] state:

> It is no coincidence that physicians who have faced their most human limitations and endured struggles similar to that of their patients return to the same message: doctors are humans too, and illness is a key part of the human experience. If doctors hope to accept illness in themselves, the profession must create an understanding and awareness of how to approach personal illness. We need to teach these skills to our students. In postgraduate education, we need to use physician narratives to inform and challenge beliefs and talk about how resilience is not a tool to overcome personal illness. These narratives are beginning to introduce a dialogue that acknowledges illness, explores how to recognise illness and to seek help, and how to support colleagues who may be facing difficulty. Doctors' accounts of their own illnesses remind health professionals and wider society that we are all human and that we are not alone when we are unwell.

Narratives, once again, are the vehicles of healing, education, and development. Issues of student, resident, and practitioner wellbeing are prevalent, a world epidemic of professional burnout has been proclaimed, and the "wounded healer" recognized.

The former five categories mostly look positively at the professional life cycle; that is, as a successful, upward trajectory that leads the novice physician to expertise, the proto-physician to maturity, and the student to seniority. These categories do not ignore the possibility of arrests and failures. Yet, they hardly dwell on these adverse personal and professional life cycle outcomes, which are sometimes temporary and constructive, but at times permanent and disabling. Nevertheless, in all categories,

---

2 Wilson, A., Millard, C., & Sabroe, I. (2019). Physician narratives of illness. *Lancet*, 394(10192), 20–21. https://doi.org/10.1016/S0140-6736(19)31501-6

accounts of illness, burnout, despair, depression, moral failure, bitterly leaving medicine, and even suicide exist.[3,4,5,6,7,8,9]

DOWNSIDES OF LIFE IN MEDICINE AND PHYSICIAN REGRETS

Additional challenges in this category include unprofessional behavior and errors. Perpetrators of breaches of professionalism have prompted the creation of the United Kingdom's General Medical Council (GMC; the agency overseeing physician performance and relicensing in the UK) in an attempt to regain public trust, and perhaps also the launch of the entire professionalism movement. In addition, the effects of inequity, prejudice, mistreatment, and abuse, often related to gender and race, are gaining visibility. Thus, the physician life cycle is also prone to ups and downs, development and disruption, whether due to breaches of professionalism, trauma, burnout, or woundedness. Indeed, looking at the doctor's trajectory from the angle of arrests in development, crises, need for remediation, or even disciplinary action, as well as "simple" ill-health, offers an additional illuminating perspective.

A study of "healthcare-related regrets" in German-speaking Switzerland reported 48 major regrets expressed by 11 physicians and 13 nurses. Each participant reported at least one regret related to a medical error, but relational issues were also prevalent. Some carried regret for up to 30 years without disclosing it. All reported a variety of troubling emotions, including

3   Rabow, M. W., Evans, C. N., & Remen, R. N. (2013). Professional formation and deformation: Repression of personal values and qualities in medical education. *Family Medicine*, *45*(1), 13–18.

4   Schwitz, F., Torti, J., & Lingard, L. (2023). What about happiness? A critical narrative review with implications for medical education. *Perspectives on Medical Education*, *12*(1), 208–217. https://doi.org/10.5334/pme.856

5   Kalet, A., & Chou, C. L. (2023). *Remediation in medical education: A mid-course correction* (2nd ed.). Springer. https://doi.org/10.1007/978-3-031-32404-8

6   Lele, K., Mclean, L. M., & Peisah, C. (2023). Beyond burnout I: Doctors health services and unmet need. *Australasian Psychiatry: Bulletin of Royal Australian and New Zealand College of Psychiatrists*, *31*(2), 139–141. https://doi.org/10.1177/10398562231159977

7   Irvine, D. (2006). A short history of the General Medical Council. *Medical Education*, *40*(3), 202–211. https://doi.org/10.1111/j.1365-2929.2006.02397.x

8   Von Arx, M., Cullati, S., Schmidt, R. E., Richner, S., Kraehenmann, R., Cheval, B., Agoritsas, T., Chopard, P., Burton-Jeangros, C., & Courvoisier, D. S. (2018). "We won't retire without skeletons in the closet": Healthcare-related regrets among physicians and nurses in German-speaking Swiss hospitals. *Qualitative Health Research*, *28*(11), 1746–1758. https://doi.org/10.1177/1049732318782434

9   Sandars, J., Patel, R., Steele, H., McAreavey, M., & Association for Medical Education Europe. (2014). Developmental student support in undergraduate medical education: AMEE Guide No. 92. *Medical Teacher*, *36*(12), 1015–1026. https://doi.org/10.3109/0142159X.2014.917166

shame, guilt, and sometimes humiliation. They also described a host of related symptoms. Coping was enhanced by what the researchers called "social capital," the cumulative support, mostly from superiors, who helped them navigate crises. Educational interventions and the modeling of processing and reflecting on trials and tribulations, emotions, and crises, is a promising modality for preventing these regrets and their disabling effects.[10,11,12]

REMEDIATION

We have already described Bebeau's approach to dentists' remediation and similar programs for physicians in the moral development category (Chapter 4). Subsequently, **Kalet** and **Chou** edited a thorough book titled *Remediation in Medical Education*,[13] now in its second edition, and published supporting papers with additional scholars.[14,15] They and many others discuss the construct of "productive failure," whereby learners' errors induce significant learning in postgraduate education (PGE), which may prompt recovery and resilience.[16,17,18,19] The book's

10 Cop, M., & Hatfield, H. (2019). Reviewing failure as part of reflection: A potential predictor of health sciences students' successes. *International Journal of Health Sciences Education*, 6(1), 1–10.

11 Kalet, A., Chou, C. L., & Ellaway, R. H. (2017). To fail is human: Remediating remediation in medical education. *Perspectives on Medical Education*, 6(6), 418–424. https://doi.org/10.1007/s40037-017-0385-6

12 Kalet, A., Guerrasio, J., & Chou, C. L. (2016). Twelve tips for developing and maintaining a remediation program in medical education. *Medical Teacher*, 38(8), 787–792. https://doi.org/10.3109/0142159X.2016.1150983

13 Kalet, A., & Chou, C. L. (2023). *Remediation in medical education: A mid-course correction* (2nd ed.). Springer. https://doi.org/10.1007/978-3-031-32404-8

14 Ellaway, R. H., Chou, C. L., & Kalet, A. L. (2018). Situating remediation: Accommodating success and failure in medical education systems. *Academic Medicine: Journal of the Association of American Medical Colleges*, 93(3), 391–398. https://doi.org/10.1097/ACM.0000000000001855

15 Chou, C. L., Kalet, A., Costa, M. J., Cleland, J., & Winston, K. (2019). Guidelines: The dos, don'ts and don't knows of remediation in medical education. *Perspectives on Medical Education*, 8(6), 322–338. https://doi.org/10.1007/s40037-019-00544-5

16 Klasen, J. M., & Lingard, L. A. (2019). Allowing failure for educational purposes in postgraduate clinical training: A narrative review. *Medical Teacher*, 41(11), 1263–1269. https://doi.org/10.1080/0142159X.2019.1630728

17 Altshuler, L., Wilhite, J. A., Hardowar, K., Crowe, R., Hanley, K., Kalet, A., Zabar, S., Gillespie, C., & Ark, T. (2023). Understanding medical student paths to communication skills expertise using latent profile analysis. *Medical Teacher*, 45(10), 1140–1147. https://doi.org/10.1080/0142159X.2023.2193303

18 Selva-Rodriguez, A., & Sandars, J. (2023). Twelve tips for providing academic remediation to widening access learners in medical education. *Medical Teacher*, 45(10), 1112–1117. https://doi.org/10.1080/0142159X.2023.2216360

19 Candilis, P. J., Kim, D. T., Sulmasy, L. S., & ACP Ethics, Professionalism and Human Rights Committee. (2019). Physician impairment and rehabilitation: Reintegration into medical practice while ensuring patient safety: A position paper from the American College of Physicians. *Annals of Internal Medicine*, 170(12), 871–879. https://doi.org/10.7326/M18-3605

many contributors describe the extensive literature on clinical errors by practicing physicians, in contrast to the relatively small number of papers identified about clinical errors by residents. Next, they display a rich gamut of approaches and practical applications to the issue at hand. There is currently a renewed interest in remediation across all stages of the physician life cycle, from student to retirement.

Two issues relevant to our review are practicing physicians' emotional responses to errors and their coping strategies after such mishaps. Scott et al.[20] report a pervasiveness of errors by health professionals: "Regardless of sex, professional background or years of experience, all participants in our study easily recalled the immediate and ongoing impact of their specific career jolting event." Overall, the intensity of the experience is influenced by the relationship between the patient and caregiver, or by past experiences. Healthcare providers are traumatized by unanticipated adverse patient events, medical error, and/or patient injury events resulting from physician error. They frequently feel so personally responsible for the patient's outcome that they become themselves a "second victim."

Scott et al. define a six-stage recovery process as follows: "(1) Chaos and accident response, (2) intrusive reflections, (3) restoring personal integrity, (4) enduring the inquisition, (5) obtaining emotional first aid and (6) moving on." These stages are sometimes intertwined, and every stage may contain coping strategies. At the third stage, "restoring personal integrity," healthcare providers seek support from a trusted individual such as a peer, supervisor, or personal confidant; seeking emotional support resembles Stage 5 of the recovery process, "obtaining emotional first aid." Disclosure of the error to family, friends, or the patient can also be interpreted as a form of coping.[21] However, a systematic review of coping with medical error found that published research does not fully bridge the gap in knowledge regarding the coping strategies of healthcare providers and those around them, including their patients. These factors may influence how clinical supervisors respond to errors by residents

20 Scott, S. D., Hirschinger, L. E., Cox, K. R., McCoig, M., Brandt, J., & Hall, L. W. (2009). The natural history of recovery for the healthcare provider "second victim" after adverse patient events. *Quality & Safety in Health Care, 18*, 325–333.

21 Sirriyeh, R., Lawton, R., Gardner, P., & Armitage, G. (2010). Coping with medical error: A systematic review of papers to assess the effects of involvement in medical errors on healthcare professionals' psychological well-being. *Quality & Safety in Health Care, 19*(6), e43. https://doi.org/10.1136/qshc.2009.035253

under their responsibility in residency teaching situations, as mentioned by **Mazor** et al.[22]

Readers may recognize that the entire simulation movement is built on the premise of providing a safe space that does not involve harm as a training ground for maintaining old skills and learning new ones.[23] In the simulation laboratory, error may be the best driver for better learning.

This is where the need for continuous deliberate practice and the master adaptive learner approach come to mind (see Chapter 3). In **Howard** and **Pusic**'s words on learning curves:

> The MAL framework explains how trainees and clinicians at all levels can improve or learn so that they can apply that learning to similar future situations. In a process known as *preparation for future learning*, a learner, ideally with the aid of an educator/coach, must invest time into learning the components of the framework. This means that in the early stages, the learner is productively double-tasked—learning the subject matter AND learning to learn. Thus, the going is initially slower than it might be otherwise; however, the learning-to-learn skills (metacognition, adaptability, approach to uncertainty) become ever more applicable moving forward, making subsequent learning easier and more effective.[24]

In aviation training, for example, a strongly statistically significant pre- to post-test improvement was observed in pilots suffering a mishap in simulation during the pre-test, regardless of the experimental group.[25]

Hauer et al. draw attention to the following:

> Despite widespread endorsement of competency-based assessment of medical trainees and practicing physicians, methods for identifying those who are not competent and strategies for remediation of

22 Mazor, K. M., Fischer, M. A., Haley, H. L., Hatem, D., & Quirk, M. E. (2005). Teaching and medical errors: Primary care preceptors' views. *Medical Education*, 39(10), 982–990. https://doi.org/10.1111/j.1365-2929.2005.02262.x

23 Guerrasio, J., & Aagaard, E. M. (2018). Long-term outcomes of a simulation-based remediation for residents and faculty with unprofessional behavior. *Journal of Graduate Medical Education*, 10(6), 693–697. https://doi.org/10.4300/JGME-D-18-00263.1

24 Howard, N., & Pusic, M. (2023). *The metacognitive competency: Becoming a master adaptive learner.* https://doi.org/10.1007/978-3-031-32404-8_4

25 Deonna, D. N., & Rhodes, W. H. (2017). Failure predicts success: Professional ethical decision-making in aviation simulators. *Journal of Character & Leadership Integration*, 4(1), 22–34. https://jcldusafa.org/index.php/jcld/article/view/176

their deficits are not standardized. … Working from these studies and research from the learning sciences, the authors propose a model that includes multiple assessment tools for identifying deficiencies, individualized instruction, deliberate practice followed by feedback and reflection, and reassessment.[26]

IMPOSTER SYNDROME, PROACTIVE QUALITY IMPROVEMENT

Studies abound about **imposter syndrome** in medicine. As **LaDonna** et al. write:

Findings from previous studies show that of participants surveyed, approximately 30% of family medicine residents (n = 175) and 44% of internal medicine residents (n = 48) feel like imposters. The imposter syndrome is a strong predictor of psychological distress; it can make physicians feel unprepared for clinical practice, and it can negatively affect their career advancement. We do not know what, if any, impact the imposter syndrome has on academic physicians' ability to both teach and support struggling learners.[27]

In addressing issues that may arise in practicing medicine, special attention is naturally paid to the remediation of unprofessional behavior[28,29] with paradigmatic, practical frameworks and a standard against which it can

26 Hauer, K. E., Ciccone, A., Henzel, T. R., Katsufrakis, P., Miller, S. H., Norcross, W. A., Papadakis, M. A., & Irby, D. M. (2009). Remediation of the deficiencies of physicians across the continuum from medical school to practice: A thematic review of the literature. *Academic Medicine: Journal of the Association of American Medical Colleges, 84*(12), 1822–1832. https://doi.org/10.1097/ACM.0b013e3181bf3170.

27 LaDonna, K. A., Ginsburg, S., & Watling, C. (2018). "Rising to the level of your incompetence": What physicians' self-assessment of their performance reveals about the imposter syndrome in medicine. *Academic Medicine: Journal of the Association of American Medical Colleges, 93*(5), 763–768. https://doi.org/10.1097/ACM .0000000000002046

28 Montgomery, M. W., Petersen, E. M., Weinstein, A. R., Curren, C., Hufmeyer, K., Kisielewski, M., Krupat, E., & Osman, N. Y. (2024). Moving beyond the dichotomous assessment of professionalism in the internal medicine clerkship: Results of a national survey of clerkship directors. *Academic Medicine: Journal of the Association of American Medical Colleges, 99*(2), 208–214. https://doi.org/10.1097/ ACM.0000000000005308

29 Norman, N. B. M., Soo, J. M. P., Lam, M. Y. K., & Thirumoorthy, T. (2021). Unprofessional behaviour of junior doctors: A retrospective analysis of outcomes by the Singapore Medical Council disciplinary tribunals. *Singapore Medical Journal, 62*(3), 120–125. https://doi.org/10.11622/smedj.2020021

be diagnosed and evaluated. Attention is also given to supporting physicians who invariably experience losses, failures, and disillusionment.[30,31] Moreover, ensuring an ongoing ethos of performance measurement, supported by data for further development and coupled with measures of wellbeing and burnout, may be the way forward. Proactively identifying potential challenges and addressing them early on, rather than only reacting when trouble occurs, may be key for physician wellbeing, productivity, and positive impact.

BACK TO THE FORTUNATE MAN

This category on physician wellbeing, illness, and mental health issues brings us back to our framing of the doctor's life cycle (DLC) through the "fortunate man," Dr. John Eskell, mentioned in the Introduction as the exemplar of British general practice in the third quarter of the last century. In subsequent publications, we learn about what was hidden in John Berger's *A Fortunate Man*: Eskell's depressive disorder, his family life (we never learn about a wife and three children in Berger's book), the calamities that he experienced after the book was published—a daughter's stroke, his wife's progressive illness and death, and the gradual decline he endured with mental illness, self-medication, deterioration of his medical competence, and eventual suicide[32]. This is not a typical story, we think. However, it is a sobering reminder of the complexity, mystery, and full spectrum of humanity of the physician's life cycle, with its overt and covert parts.

30 Bennet, G. (1987). *The wound and the doctor: Healing, technology and power in modern medicine*. Secker & Warburg.

31 Barnhoorn, P. C., Houtlosser, M., Ottenhoff-de Jonge, M. W., Essers, G. T. J. M., Numans, M. E., & Kramer, A. W. M. (2019). A practical framework for remediating unprofessional behavior and for developing professionalism competencies and a professional identity. *Medical Teacher*, 41(3), 303–308. https://doi.org/10.1080/0142159X.2018.1464133

32 O'Mahony, S. (2022). A fortunate man? *The Lancet*, 399(10332), 1129620–7. https://doi.org/10.1016/S0140-6736(22)00574-8

Summary

The opening story introduces how a physician experiences personal serious health trouble, a sobering instance that invariably summons deep reflection on life, uncertainty, and the profession. This category sheds light on the darker, yet inevitable, side of the physician's life cycle, where ill-health and woundedness, as well as error, unprofessional behavior, failure, imposter syndrome, shame, and regret exist. Coupled with potential moral distress and injury described in the moral development category (Chapter 4), the imperative of confronting one's difficulties and leaving the comfort zone—as described in all the categories, almost as a precondition for progress—makes us aware of how formidable the risks and trials on the journey are. Here, issues of character and resilience building when remediation is necessary come to mind. The ethos of imperfection mentioned in the previous category looms large in the present one. Once again, we reiterate that most physicians do not reach their full potential. In this category, a view of the many obstacles to mastery and flourishing is presented along with optional mechanisms to navigate them. With the tragic unfolding of the Fortunate Man described in the closing paragraph as a cautionary tale, there is reason to believe that even with severe ill-health, serious error, and perceived failure, ongoing development throughout the life cycle is possible with skillful and effective remediation and support, enabling the recovered practitioner to regain the option for transformation.

REFERENCES

Altshuler, L., Wilhite, J. A., Hardowar, K., Crowe, R., Hanley, K., Kalet, A., Zabar, S., Gillespie, C., & Ark, T. (2023). Understanding medical student paths to communication skills expertise using latent profile analysis. *Medical Teacher*, 45(10), 1140–1147. https://doi.org/10.1080/0142159X.2023.2193303

Barnhoorn, P. C., Houtlosser, M., Ottenhoff-de Jonge, M. W., Essers, G. T. J. M., Numans, M. E., & Kramer, A. W. M. (2019). A practical framework for remediating unprofessional behavior and for developing professionalism competencies and a professional identity. *Medical Teacher*, 41(3), 303–308. https://doi.org/10.1000/0142159X.2018.1464133

Bennet, G. (1987). *The wound and the doctor: Healing, technology and power in modern medicine*. Secker & Warburg.

Candilis, P. J., Kim, D. T., Sulmasy, L. S., & ACP Ethics, Professionalism and Human Rights Committee. (2019). Physician impairment and rehabilitation: Reintegration into medical practice while ensuring patient safety: A position paper from the American College of Physicians. *Annals of Internal Medicine*, 170(12), 871–879. https://doi.org/10.7326/M18-3605

Chou, C. L., Kalet, A., Costa, M. J., Cleland, J., & Winston, K. (2019). Guidelines: The dos, don'ts and don't knows of remediation in medical education. *Perspectives on Medical Education*, 8(6), 322–338. https://doi.org/10.1007/s40037-019-00544-5

Cop, M., & Hatfield, H. (2019). Reviewing failure as part of reflection: A potential predictor of health sciences students' successes. *International Journal of Health Sciences Education*, 6(1), 1–10.

Deonna, D. N., & Rhodes, W. H. (2017). Failure predicts success: Professional ethical decision-making in aviation simulators. *Journal of Character & Leadership Integration*, 4(1), 22–34. https://jcldusafa.org/index.php/jcld/article/view/176

Ellaway, R. H., Chou, C. L., & Kalet, A. L. (2018). Situating remediation: Accommodating success and failure in medical education systems. *Academic Medicine: Journal of the Association of American Medical Colleges*, 93(3), 391–398. https://doi.org/10.1097/ACM.0000000000001855

Guerrasio, J., & Aagaard, E. M. (2018). Long-term outcomes of a simulation-based remediation for residents and faculty with unprofessional behavior. *Journal of Graduate Medical Education*, 10(6), 693–697. https://doi.org/10.4300/JGME-D-18-00263.1

Hauer, K. E., Ciccone, A., Henzel, T. R., Katsufrakis, P., Miller, S. H., Norcross, W. A., Papadakis, M. A., & Irby, D. M. (2009). Remediation of the deficiencies of physicians across the continuum from medical school to practice: A thematic review of the literature. *Academic Medicine: Journal of the Association of American Medical Colleges*, 84(12), 1822–1832. https://doi.org/10.1097/ACM.0b013e3181bf3170

Howard, N., & Pusic, M. (2023). *The metacognitive competency: Becoming a master adaptive learner.* https://doi.org/10.1007/978-3-031-32404-8_4

Irvine, D. (2006). A short history of the General Medical Council. *Medical Education*, 40(3), 202–211. https://doi.org/10.1111/j.1365-2929.2006.02397.x

Kalet, A., & Chou, C. L. (2023). *Remediation in medical education: A mid-course correction* (2nd ed.). Springer. https://doi.org/10.1007/978-3-031-32404-8

Kalet, A., Chou, C. L., & Ellaway, R. H. (2017). To fail is human: Remediating remediation in medical education. *Perspectives on Medical Education*, 6(6), 418–424. https://doi.org/10.1007/s40037-017-0385-6

Kalet, A., Guerrasio, J., & Chou, C. L. (2016). Twelve tips for developing and maintaining a remediation program in medical education. *Medical Teacher*, 38(8), 787–792. https://doi.org/10.3109/0142159X.2016.1150983

Klasen, J. M., & Lingard, L. A. (2019). Allowing failure for educational purposes in postgraduate clinical training: A narrative review. *Medical Teacher*, 41(11), 1263–1269. https://doi.org/10.1080/0142159X.2019.1630728

LaDonna, K. A., Ginsburg, S., & Watling, C. (2018). "Rising to the level of your incompetence": What physicians' self-assessment of their performance reveals about the imposter syndrome in medicine. *Academic Medicine: Journal of the Association of American Medical Colleges*, 93(5), 763–768. https://doi.org/10.1097/ACM.0000000000002046

Lele, K., Mclean, L. M., & Peisah, C. (2023). Beyond burnout I: Doctors health services and unmet need. *Australasian Psychiatry: Bulletin of Royal Australian and New Zealand College of Psychiatrists*, 31(2), 139–141. https://doi.org/10.1177/10398562231159977

Mazor, K. M., Fischer, M. A., Haley, H. L., Hatem, D., & Quirk, M. E. (2005). Teaching and medical errors: Primary care preceptors' views. *Medical Education*, 39(10), 982–990. https://doi.org/10.1111/j.1365-2929.2005.02262.x

Montgomery, M. W., Petersen, E. M., Weinstein, A. R., Curren, C., Hufmeyer, K., Kisielewski, M., Krupat, E., & Osman, N. Y. (2024). Moving beyond the dichotomous assessment of professionalism in the internal medicine clerkship: Results of a national survey of clerkship directors. *Academic Medicine: Journal of the Association of American Medical Colleges*, 99(2), 208–214. https://doi.org/10.1097/ACM.0000000000005308

Norman, N. B. M., Soo, J. M. P., Lam, M. Y. K., & Thirumoorthy, T. (2021). Unprofessional behaviour of junior doctors: A retrospective analysis of outcomes by the Singapore Medical Council disciplinary tribunals. *Singapore Medical Journal*, 62(3), 120–125. https://doi.org/10.11622/smedj.2020021

O'Mahony, S. (2022). A fortunate man? *The Lancet*, 399(10332), 1129620–7. https://doi.org/10.1016/S0140-6736(22)00574-8

Rabow, M. W., Evans, C. N., & Remen, R. N. (2013). Professional formation and deformation: Repression of personal values and qualities in medical education. *Family Medicine*, 45(1), 13–18.

Sandars, J., Patel, R., Steele, H., McAreavey, M., & Association for Medical Education Europe. (2014). Developmental student support in undergraduate medical education: AMEE Guide No. 92. *Medical Teacher*, 36(12), 1015–1026. https://doi.org/10.3109/0142159X.2014.917166

Schwitz, F., Torti, J., & Lingard, L. (2023). What about happiness? A critical narrative review with implications for medical education. *Perspectives on Medical Education*, 12(1), 208–217. https://doi.org/10.5334/pme.856

Scott, S. D., Hirschinger, L. E., Cox, K. R., McCoig, M., Brandt, J., & Hall, L. W. (2009). The natural history of recovery for the healthcare provider "second victim" after adverse patient events. *Quality & Safety in Health Care*, 18, 325–333.

Selva-Rodriguez, A., & Sandars, J. (2023). Twelve tips for providing academic remediation to widening access learners in medical education. *Medical Teacher*, 45(10), 1112–1117. https://doi.org/10.1080/0142159X.2023.2216360

Sirriyeh, R., Lawton, R., Gardner, P., & Armitage, G. (2010). Coping with medical error: A systematic review of papers to assess the effects of involvement in medical errors on healthcare professionals' psychological well-being. *Quality & Safety in Health Care*, 19(6), e43. https://doi.org/10.1136/qshc.2009.035253

Von Arx, M., Cullati, S., Schmidt, R. E., Richner, S., Kraehenmann, R., Cheval, B., Agoritsas, T., Chopard, P., Burton-Jeangros, C., & Courvoisier, D. S. (2018). "We won't retire without skeletons in the closet": Healthcare-related regrets among physicians and nurses in German-speaking Swiss hospitals. *Qualitative Health Research*, 28(11), 1746–1758. https://doi.org/10.1177/1049732318782434

Weston, W. W. Unpublished personal narrative.

Wilson, A., Millard, C., & Sabroe, I. (2019). Physician narratives of illness. *Lancet*, 394(10192), 20–21. https://doi.org/10.1016/S0140-6736(19)31501-6

Gender, race, and core identities

Bias, discrimination, and mistreatment in medicine

....

A horse of a different color

Soon after arriving in the *Goldene Medine*,* my shoelaces started falling apart. They must have been cheap stuff. I asked Noa, my wife, to find a replacement. Not for me, but for the shoelaces. I didn't have the mental space or time to search for the precisely right ones. Close but no cigar. She tried her best, but what she procured was not quite right, yet they had to do. Traveling the country with untidy shoelaces, unbuttoned top shirt button, sans tie, was the casual Israeli "ok" image I continue to curate to this day.

I also struggled with THE LOOKS that came my way in the stores, gas stations, or odd offices when I opened my mouth to speak. It was my accent, I guess, the guttural, raw, and very foreign accent of a Hebrew speaker. Sometimes I needed to repeat myself three or four times on the phone before I could get my message across. At the beginning of my tenure as a visiting family medicine professor, shadowing in the family medicine clinic (usually fly-on-the-wall style), I'd get puzzled looks from patients when I began speaking. The doctor I was accompanying, the one I was teaching, needed to give me a hand. I sizzled with paranoia—America must be full of antisemites, xenophobes, and racists, I thought.

This unsettled me, which was unlike me. I needed to get to work. So, I started listening. Really listening.

---

* Goldene Medine—Yiddish for "Golden Country," a common description of the United States by Jewish immigrants, especially in the late 19th and early 20th centuries.

DOI: 10.1201/9781003507529-8

Early on, I discovered that the local dialect is half idiomatic English, the other half slang. Placing my bets on the first, I diligently recorded each idiom that came up in conversations in my new bible, a CVS memo pad. I was convinced it would cost me an arm and a leg, but sharing these precious collected phrases with my colleagues and friends was rewarded with smiles, chuckles, and a warm glow of acceptance.

Some idioms were quite handy. They enabled me to dance to my own music, square things up, and kept me on top of the game. Stepping up to the plate of Red Sox Nation lingo and nonchalantly dropping expressions like "curveballs" or "pitch in," I quickly sensed I was earning some serious mileage in New England. Various expressions, however, threw me way off kilter, requiring some labor-intensive Googling to decipher their meaning and origins. I was out on a limb with, for example, "more honored in the breach than the observance" (from *Hamlet*, Act 1, Scene IV). But, hey, cut me some slack, I learned that Shakespeare meant "better broken than observed," not "more often broken than observed"! Can't shoot from the hip with this stuff. …

Emailing the results of my diligent search to a highly respected professor, I scored a few points. Halfway through the year, with many irons in the fire, I encountered this fellow by chance. He strode into a room in which I was having a conversation with three other colleagues. When I spoke, he gave me THE LOOK. Head tilted slightly to one side, eyes narrowed, forehead crinkled with that "why do I have to tolerate these strangers and their abuse of my language" frown. I was pretty sure, then and there, that this must be a highly educated bigot. I made sure that I got a chance to respectfully confront him at a later point in time and even the score. Alas, I was humbled by what transpired: this colleague, I discovered, was hard of hearing. THE LOOK was a tilt of the head that puts the better ear forward; the frown was the intense effort to make sense of an unusual accent, made much more difficult given the background noise. It is never too late to apologize.

Now nearing the end of my sabbatical year, it is almost smooth sailing. I'm not sure exactly why. With paranoia markedly diminished, I more easily weather the less threatening "looks" and frowns that continue to greet my deeply entrenched accent. Hey, it's almost a piece of cake. Am I broken in? It is a relief to no longer walk on eggshells, nor bend over backwards to belong. I now easily find my way around town; even New York and Boston are not intimidating anymore.

The other day in South Station I noticed a "Shoe and Luggage Repair" sign. I entered the melting pot: two fellow non-natives—sporting accents, darker skin color, and command of what sounded like an African language—were very helpful. I purchased two pairs of prim and proper black and brown shoelaces, the cat's meow. Cutting to the chase, my old, badly worn shoelaces have been unceremoniously discarded. It is as if I am now cooking with gas. It feels right: my shoes at least look like they belong. No necktie yet, so I fasten the top shirt button more often. Even though it seems like throwing a deck chair off the *Queen Mary*, or rearranging similar ones on the *Titanic*, this has made a difference. (These idioms are my favorites so far.)

Lo and behold, on a recent visit to the Pawtucket Slater Mill, I learned that Rhode Island was once the shoelace capital of the United States. As the end of my year in America, the *Goldene Medine*, draws near, I almost feel at home. Occasionally even my accent is mellowing, and English feels almost natural. Ah, the icing on the cake. For all the tea in China I won't take "accent reduction" classes nor will I enroll in "THE LOOK avoidance academy." I was barking up the wrong tree, wasn't I? I will settle on proposing an idiomatic English institute to my liking. The final exam will feature a shoelace-matching exercise. Let's get the ball rolling.[1]

* * *

The opening story, a humorous one for a change, gives voice to experiencing otherness around a foreign accent and idiosyncratic idioms. While we have addressed individual adverse aspects that may arise throughout the doctor's life cycle (DLC) in Chapter 6, including woundedness and the need for remediation, in this category we direct our gaze to the structural ones. The issues presented in both categories have not attracted widespread attention or visibility in the past. However, in the last decade and especially the last few years, they have been assuming a much more central role in the professional discourse, along with the next category (Chapter 8), which is focused on the impact of the coronavirus pandemic.[2,3,4] A significant shift is taking place, from a landscape of maximizing the physician's potential to a much deeper delve into possible obstacles on the path to this noble goal.

Our inquiry has identified the following components of the present category:

---

1   Reis, S. P. (2008). A horse of a different color. Personal communication.

2   Simpson, D., Bidwell, J., La Fratta, T., & Agard, K. (2022). Using a milestone framework for assessing resident, fellow, and faculty competence in diversity, equity, and inclusion. *Journal of Graduate Medical Education*, *14*(3), 342–343. https://doi.org/10.4300/JGME-D-21-00940.1

3   Wyatt, T. R., Rockich-Winston, N., White, D., & Taylor, T. R. (2021). "Changing the narrative": A study on professional identity formation among Black/African American physicians in the U.S. *Advances in Health Sciences Education: Theory and Practice*, *26*(1), 183–198. https://doi.org/10.1007/s10459-020-09978-7

4   Crampton, P. E. S., & Afzali, Y. (2021). Professional identity formation, intersectionality and equity in medical education. *Medical Education*, *55*(2), 140–142. https://doi.org/10.1111/medu.14415

1. **Gender** is a major factor in personal and professional development. Women still have a radically different trajectory with gender-specific inequity in multiple dimensions, adversely affecting their evolving identities, careers, and wellbeing.[5,6,7,8,9,10,11,12,13]

2. **Race and ethnicity,** as well as a myriad of additional core minority identities, also radically shape the developmental journey.[14]

5   Pelley, E., & Carnes, M. (2020). When a specialty becomes "women's work": Trends in and implications of specialty gender segregation in medicine. *Academic Medicine: Journal of the Association of American Medical Colleges, 95*(10), 1499–1506. https://doi.org/10.1097/ACM.0000000000003555

6   Haggins, A. N. (2020). To be seen, heard, and valued: Strategies to promote a sense of belonging for women and underrepresented in medicine physicians. *Academic Medicine: Journal of the Association of American Medical Colleges, 95*(10), 1507–1510. https://doi.org/10.1097/ACM.0000000000003553

7   Helzer, E. G., Myers, C. G., Fahim, C., Sutcliffe, K. M., & Abernathy, J. H. (2020). Gender bias in collaborative medical decision making: Emergent evidence. *Academic Medicine: Journal of the Association of American Medical Colleges, 95*(10), 1524–1528. https://doi.org/10.1097/ACM.0000000000003590

8   Barnes, K. L., Dunivan, G., Sussman, A. L., McGuire, L., & McKee, R. (2020). Behind the mask: An exploratory assessment of female surgeons' experiences of gender bias. *Academic Medicine: Journal of the Association of American Medical Colleges, 95*(10), 1529–1538. https://doi.org/10.1097/ACM.0000000000003569

9   Manne-Goehler, J., Freund, K. M., Raj, A., Kaplan, S. E., Terrin, N., Breeze, J. L., & Carr, P. L. (2020). Evaluating the role of self-esteem on differential career outcomes by gender in academic medicine. *Academic Medicine: Journal of the Association of American Medical Colleges, 95*(10), 1558–1562. https://doi.org/10.1097/ACM .0000000000003138

10 Stack, S. W., Jagsi, R., Biermann, J. S., Lundberg, G. P., Law, K. L., Milne, C. K., Williams, S. G., Burton, T. C., Larison, C. L., & Best, J. A. (2020). Childbearing decisions in residency: A multicenter survey of female residents. *Academic Medicine: Journal of the Association of American Medical Colleges, 95*(10), 1550–1557. https:// doi.org/10.1097/ACM.0000000000003549

11 Periyakoil, V. S., Chaudron, L., Hill, E. V., Pellegrini, V., Neri, E., & Kraemer, H. C. (2020). Common types of gender-based microaggressions in medicine. *Academic Medicine: Journal of the Association of American Medical Colleges, 95*(3), 450–457. https://doi.org/10.1097/ACM.0000000000003057

12 Rogers, A. C., Wren, S. M., & McNamara, D. A. (2019). Gender and specialty influences on personal and professional life among trainees. *Annals of Surgery, 269*(2), 383–387. https://doi.org/10.1097/SLA.0000000000002580

13 Barnes, K. L., McGuire, L., Dunivan, G., Sussman, A. L., & McKee, R. (2019). Gender bias experiences of female surgical trainees. *Journal of Surgical Education, 76*(6), e1–e14. https://doi.org/10.1016/j.jsurg.2019.07.024

14 Wyatt, T. R., Rockich-Winston, N., Taylor, T. R., & White, D. (2020). What does context have to do with anything? A study of professional identity formation in physician-trainees considered underrepresented in medicine. *Academic Medicine: Journal of the Association of American Medical Colleges, 95*(10), 1587–1593. https://doi.org /10.1097/ACM.0000000000003192

3. **Bias, discrimination, macro- and microaggressions** challenge growth and inflict suffering and disadvantage.[15,16] Mistreatment and even occasional abuse across hierarchical structures (i.e., student, resident, subordinate), independent of or in conjunction with the above two items, are ubiquitous.[17,18]

While the professional community is increasingly shedding light on these recesses of the professional experience and committing to abolishing them and assuring universal structural competence, their deep-rooted effects are still widespread and unfortunately disabling.[19] They are associated with the inherent risk of abuse of power in medicine (see Chapters 4 and 5), albeit this time directed within the profession and not only toward patients.

GENDER

Lockyer et al. write:

> Being a woman and a physician can influence career consolidation and professional identity as a physician. ... While the last fifty years have witnessed a tremendous increase in the proportion of women in full-time work ... female physicians with children are less likely to work full time than their male counterparts with children ... providing or managing care for elderly parents or disabled spouses.[20]

---

15 Torres, M. B., Salles, A., & Cochran, A. (2019). Recognizing and reacting to microaggressions in medicine and surgery. *JAMA Surgery, 154*(9), 868–872. https://doi.org/10.1001/jamasurg.2019.1648

16 Molina, M. F., Landry, A. I., Chary, A. N., & Burnett-Bowie, S. M. (2020). Addressing the elephant in the room: Microaggressions in medicine. *Annals of Emergency Medicine, 76*(4), 387–391. https://doi.org/10.1016/j.annemergmed.2020.04.009

17 Fnais, N., Soobiah, C., Chen, M. H., Lillie, E., Perrier, L., Tashkhandi, M., Straus, S. E., Mamdani, M., Al-Omran, M., & Tricco, A. C. (2014). Harassment and discrimination in medical training: A systematic review and meta-analysis. *Academic Medicine: Journal of the Association of American Medical Colleges, 89*(5), 817–827. https://doi.org/10.1097/ACM.0000000000000200

18 Hoskison, K., & Beasley, B. W. (2019). A conversation about the role of humiliation in teaching: The ugly, the bad, and the good. *Academic Medicine: Journal of the Association of American Medical Colleges, 94*(8), 1078–1080. https://doi.org/10.1097/ACM.0000000000002594

19 Chen. D. R., & Priest, K. (2019). Pimping: A tradition of gendered disempowerment. *BMC Medical Education, 19*(1), 345. https://doi.org/10.1186/s12909-019-1761-1

20 Lockyer, J., de Groot, J., & Silver, I. (2016). Professional identity formation, the practicing physician and continuing professional development. In R. L. Cruess, S. R. Cruess, & Y. Steinert (Eds.), *Teaching medical professionalism: Supporting the development of a professional identity* (pp. 186–200). Cambridge University Press.

Roberts[21] provides a detailed account of the following facts: in the United States, while highly represented in the nation's gender composition in basic medical education (BME), graduate medical education (GME), and the lower ranks of academic and clinical pursuits, "women continue to be underrepresented in top leadership roles in academic medicine" and are "rarely appointed to oversee high-stakes and highly influential clinical or research missions." They are disadvantaged in promotion, R01 grant acquisition, institutional research support, professional and scientific journal editor positions, and scientific publications. Furthermore, "mentors to help women faculty deal with such challenges appear to be in short supply," and female presence in academic medicine is still a "revolving door" with many leaving the field due to multiple barriers.

In addition to facing the proverbial glass ceiling, "half of women in medical school have experienced sexual harassment, most commonly gender-based harassment, and even more women faculty, cumulatively, have these experiences across the course of their careers in medicine."

Women must work harder for academic recognition, experience "an incident of overt disrespect" at a rate 17 times higher than that of their male counterparts, and report "more severe, frequent, and stressful microaggressions." This unsupportive culture undermines their success and increases life–work conflicts. Societal expectations still require of women greater involvement in their homes, thus increasing "role strain and stress." On average, women spend 8.5 more hours weekly performing "domestic" activities than their male spouses with a similar career. They are also more likely to take time off work when their children are ill or when a disruption of childcare services occurs, a trend widely amplified during the COVID-19 pandemic.[22]

Consequently, women in medicine experience greater fatigue, burnout, and adverse physical and mental health outcomes, including "a significantly higher suicide risk" for female physicians relative to male physicians and women in the general population.[23] Moreover, they are disadvantaged in their remuneration in both academia and practice.

---

21 Roberts, L. W. (2020). Women and academic medicine, 2020. *Academic Medicine: Journal of the Association of American Medical Colleges, 95*(10), 1459–1464. https://doi.org/10.1097/ACM.0000000000003617

22 Chen, I., & Bougie, O. (2020). Women's issues in pandemic times: How COVID-19 has exacerbated gender inequities for women in Canada and around the world. *Journal of Obstetrics and Gynaecology Canada (JOGC), 42*(12), 1458. https://doi.org/10.1016/j.jogc.2020.06.010

23 Duarte, D., El-Hagrassy, M. M., Couto, T. C. E., Gurgel, W., Fregni, F., & Correa, H. (2020). Male and female physician suicidality: A systematic review and meta-analysis. *JAMA Psychiatry, 77*(6), 587–597. https://doi.org/10.1001/jamapsychiatry.2020.0011

A special concern is the experience of female residents, especially in surgical specialties, regarding pregnancy, childbearing, and parenting.[24,25,26] These include disproportionate infertility, pregnancy complications, and negative outcomes, as well as stress around "heteronormative expectations of women in medicine—for example, to be married to members of the opposite sex, to have children, or to be capable of healthy pregnancies—[which] can contribute to the feeling of being different, excluded, and/or of not belonging."

Needless to say, the resulting life cycle for female physicians may significantly differ from that of their male counterparts. This reality calls for a positive transformation of policies, procedures, and deep-seated inequities to allow for a radically better and just experience.

RACE, ETHNICITY, AND UNDERREPRESENTED IDENTITIES

Having a racial or ethnic identity that differs from the dominant one, such as being Black or Latino in North America or having a foreign accent, as the opening narrative of this category illustrates, radically shapes the developmental experience for these physicians. This issue has gained increasing recognition in health professions education and healthcare, especially following the momentum gained by the Black Lives Matter movement in the United States and the striking disparities highlighted by the COVID-19 pandemic.[27]

Other minority or stigmatized identities suffer the same fate. These include sexual orientation and gender identities (such as LGBTQIA+), religious affiliation (differing from the dominant religion, especially if it has a visible external expression), and special needs or disabilities, to

24 Todd, A. R., Cawthorn, T. R., & Temple-Oberle, C. (2020). Pregnancy and parenthood remain challenging during surgical residency: A systematic review. *Academic Medicine: Journal of the Association of American Medical Colleges*, 95(10), 1607–1615. https://doi.org/10.1097/ACM.0000000000003351

25 Stack, S. W., McKinney, C. M., Spiekerman, C., & Best, J. A. (2018). Childbearing and maternity leave in residency: Determinants and well-being outcomes. *Postgraduate Medical Journal*, 94(1118), 694–699. https://doi.org/10.1136/postgradmedj-2018-135960

26 Stack, S. W., Eurich, K. E., Kaplan, E. A., Ball, A. L., Mookherjee, S., & Best, J. A. (2019). Parenthood during graduate medical education: A scoping review. *Academic Medicine: Journal of the Association of American Medical Colleges*, 94(11), 1814–1824. https://doi.org/10.1097/ACM.0000000000002948

27 Sukhera, J., Kulkarni, C., & Taylor, T. (2021). Structural distress: Experiences of moral distress related to structural stigma during the COVID-19 pandemic. *Perspectives on Medical Education*, 10(4), 222–229. https://doi.org/10.1007/s40037-021-00663-y

name a few.[28,29] These challenges are further compounded for women. Thus, "women and men who identify as underrepresented in medicine (URiM) have reported racial bias in the form of microaggressions, othering, and extra workplace burdens that contribute considerably to workplace stress reported in many studies." Minority health professionals also perceive current constructs such as professionalism as restrictive and potentially oppressive and seek their constructive adaptations.[30]

Healthcare and health professions education have responded to this discriminatory reality with the diversity, equity, and inclusion (DEI) movement.[31] It is most visible in North America and is operationalized through multiple governance, curricular, and social interventions.[32] Of note are interventions to activate bystanders to become upstanders, connecting this category with the moral development one (Chapter 4). Recently, fueled by the war in Gaza, hate speech and activities have grown exponentially, with a particular increase in rhetoric and incidents targeting Jewish students and faculty.[33] Current criticism that DEI has neglected to include antisemitism as a threat to equity and inclusion is challenging.[34]

28 Woodford, M. R., Howell, M. L., Kulick, A., & Silverschanz, P. (2013). "That's so gay": Heterosexual male undergraduates and the perpetuation of sexual orientation microaggressions on campus. *Journal of Interpersonal Violence*, 28(2), 416–435. https://doi.org/10.1177/0886260512454719

29 Lee, E. J., Ditchman, N., Thomas, J., & Tsen, J. (2019). Microaggressions experienced by people with multiple sclerosis in the workplace: An exploratory study using Sue's taxonomy. *Rehabilitation Psychology*, 64(2), 179–193. https://doi.org/10.1037/rep0000269

30 Maristany, D., Hauer, K. E., Leep Hunderfund, A. N., Elks, M. L., Bullock, J. L., Kumbamu, A., & O'Brien, B. C. (2023). The problem and power of professionalism: A critical analysis of medical students' and residents' perspectives and experiences of professionalism. *Academic Medicine: Journal of the Association of American Medical Colleges*, 98(11S), S32–S41. https://doi.org/10.1097/ACM.0000000000005367

31 Wei, C., Bernstein, S. A., Gu, A., Mehta, A., Sharma, D., Mortman, R., Verduzco-Gutierrez, M., & Chretien, K. C. (2023). Evaluating diversity and inclusion content on graduate medical education websites. *Journal of General Internal Medicine*, 38(3), 582–585. https://doi.org/10.1007/s11606-022-07973-9

32 Tyson, L., Skinner, J., Hariharan, B., Josiah, B., Okongwu, K., & Semlyen, J. (2024). Tackling discrimination in medicine head on: The impact of bystander intervention training. *Medical Teacher*, 1–10. Advance online publication. https://doi.org/10.1080/0142159X.2024.2316849

33 French, D. (2024, January 14). Opinion | This is the actual danger posed by D.E.I. *New York Times* (nytimes.com). Accessed September 7, 2024.

34 Asare, J. G. (2023, July 20). Is DEI officially dead? Forbes.com. Accessed September 7, 2024.

MISTREATMENT AND ABUSE

In addition to the bias and discrimination described earlier in this chapter, reports of widespread mistreatment and abuse in medical education and practice abound.[35] Frequent manifestations of mistreatment include: "pimping" (an abrasive questioning style),[36] microaggressions (often related to gender or race), neglect,[37] unfair treatment and demands,[38] and inattention to basic psychological and physical needs.[39,40] These occur in educational settings where senior supervisors and teachers sometimes humiliate juniors, and in the workplace where bullying, maltreatment, and abuse are prevalent. Such adverse experiences may result in shame, guilt, anxiety and depression, scholastic and practice failure, and ill-health. Further, recent literature suggests that perceived "unprofessional" behavior results from such abuse.

Interventions are being offered to address this concerning reality. **Trauma-informed medical education and care** are being promoted, with the view that the consequences of abuse and mistreatment should be recognized as potentially traumatic, and that attention to past personal adverse events should be incorporated into care and curricula.[41,42,43]

35 Reifler, D. (2016). Pimping as a practice in medical education—Reply. *JAMA*, *315*(20), 2237. https://doi.org/10.1001/jama.2016.1582

36 Reifler, D. R. (2015). The pedagogy of pimping: Educational rigor or mistreatment? *JAMA*, *314*(22), 2355–2356. https://doi.org/10.1001/jama.2015.14670

37 Romanski, P. A., Bartz, D., Pelletier, A., & Johnson, N. R. (2020). The "invisible student": Neglect as a form of medical student mistreatment, a call to action. *Journal of Surgical Education*, *77*(6), 1327–1330. https://doi.org/10.1016/j.jsurg.2020.05.013

38 Dyrbye, L. N., West, C. P., Herrin, J., Dovidio, J., Cunningham, B., Yeazel, M., Lam, V., Onyeador, I. N., Wittlin, N. M., Burke, S. E., Hayes, S. N., Phelan, S. M., & van Ryn, M. (2021). A longitudinal study exploring learning environment culture and subsequent risk of burnout among resident physicians overall and by gender. *Mayo Clinic Proceedings*, *96*(8), 2168–2183. https://doi.org/10.1016/j.mayocp.2020.12.036

39 Sharifi, M., Asadi-Pooya, A. A., & Mousavi-Roknabadi, R. S. (2020). Burnout among healthcare providers of COVID-19; A systematic review of epidemiology and recommendations. *Archives of Academic Emergency Medicine*, *9*(1), e7. https://doi.org/10.22037/aaem.v9i1.1004

40 Chaudhri, S., Zweig, K. C., Hebbar, P., Angell, S., & Vasan, A. (2019). Trauma-informed care: A strategy to improve primary healthcare engagement for persons with criminal justice system involvement. *Journal of General Internal Medicine*, *34*(6), 1048–1052. https://doi.org/10.1007/s11606-018-4783-1

41 Trauma-Informed Care Toolkit | Center to Advance Palliative Care (capc.org).

42 Elisseou, S., Puranam, S., & Nandi, M. (2018). A novel, trauma-informed physical examination curriculum. *Medical Education*, *52*(5), 555–556. https://doi.org/10.1111/medu.13569

43 Biggs, L., Cosey-Gay, F., Dinizulu, S. M., Harper, D., King, J., Mitchell, A., Pines, M., Rogers, S. O., Jr., & Stolbach, B. (2023). Improving trauma-informed care in the

Summary

In the past, only scant attention was paid to how determinants of adversity in the DLC impact the personal and professional developmental trajectories of women and minorities. This is now radically changing, as the discourse of medical education in the current decade, especially in the wake of the coronavirus and racism epidemics, has catalyzed diversity, equity, and inclusion (DEI) initiatives. Adversity related to bias, discrimination, and harassment, overlapping with the previous two categories, further impedes the flourishing of professional identity formation. Educational interventions to address these challenges are multiplying, yet still at times fall short of being sufficiently effective and inclusive. As already mentioned, this category is a daunting challenge that is shaking the foundations of former norms and discourses. Thus, as we move forward in this inquiry, the going gets harder.

REFERENCES

Asare, J. G. (2023, July 20). Is DEI officially dead? Forbes.com. Accessed September 7, 2024.

Barnes, K. L., Dunivan, G., Sussman, A. L., McGuire, L., & McKee, R. (2020). Behind the mask: An exploratory assessment of female surgeons' experiences of gender bias. *Academic Medicine: Journal of the Association of American Medical Colleges*, 95(10), 1529–1538. https://doi.org/10.1097/ACM.0000000000003569

Barnes, K. L., McGuire, L., Dunivan, G., Sussman, A. L., & McKee, R. (2019). Gender bias experiences of female surgical trainees. *Journal of Surgical Education*, 76(6), e1–e14. https://doi.org/10.1016/j.jsurg.2019.07.024

Biggs, L., Cosey-Gay, F., Dinizulu, S. M., Harper, D., King, J., Mitchell, A., Pines, M., Rogers, S. O., Jr., & Stolbach, B. (2023). Improving trauma-informed care in the face of firearm violence. *New England Journal of Medicine*, 389(20), e40. https://doi.org/10.1056/NEJMp2310060

Chaudhri, S., Zweig, K. C., Hebbar, P., Angell, S., & Vasan, A. (2019). Trauma-informed care: A strategy to improve primary healthcare engagement for persons with criminal justice system involvement. *Journal of General Internal Medicine*, 34(6), 1048–1052. https://doi.org/10.1007/s11606-018-4783-1

Chen, D. R., & Priest, K. (2019). Pimping: A tradition of gendered disempowerment. *BMC Medical Education*, 19(1), 345. https://doi.org/10.1186/s12909-019-1761-1

Chen, I., & Bougie, O. (2020). Women's issues in pandemic times: How COVID-19 has exacerbated gender inequities for women in Canada and around the world. *Journal of Obstetrics and Gynaecology Canada (JOGC)*, 42(12), 1458. https://doi.org/10.1016/j.jogc.2020.06.010

Crampton, P. E. S., & Afzali, Y. (2021). Professional identity formation, intersectionality and equity in medical education. *Medical Education*, 55(2), 140–142. https://doi.org/10.1111/medu.14415

face of firearm violence. *New England Journal of Medicine*, 389(20), e40. https://doi.org/10.1056/NEJMp2310060

Duarte, D., El-Hagrassy, M. M., Couto, T. C. E., Gurgel, W., Fregni, F., & Correa, H. (2020). Male and female physician suicidality: A systematic review and meta-analysis. *JAMA Psychiatry*, 77(6), 587–597. https://doi.org/10.1001/jamapsychiatry .2020.0011

Dyrbye, L. N., West, C. P., Herrin, J., Dovidio, J., Cunningham, B., Yeazel, M., Lam, V., Onyeador, I. N., Wittlin, N. M., Burke, S. E., Hayes, S. N., Phelan, S. M., & van Ryn, M. (2021). A longitudinal study exploring learning environment culture and subsequent risk of burnout among resident physicians overall and by gender. *Mayo Clinic Proceedings*, 96(8), 2168–2183. https://doi.org/10.1016/j.mayocp.2020 .12.036

Elisseou, S., Puranam, S., & Nandi, M. (2018). A novel, trauma-informed physical examination curriculum. *Medical Education*, 52(5), 555–556. https://doi.org/10 .1111/medu.13569

Fnais, N., Soobiah, C., Chen, M. H., Lillie, E., Perrier, L., Tashkhandi, M., Straus, S. E., Mamdani, M., Al-Omran, M., & Tricco, A. C. (2014). Harassment and discrimination in medical training: A systematic review and meta-analysis. *Academic Medicine: Journal of the Association of American Medical Colleges*, 89(5), 817–827. https://doi.org/10.1097/ACM.0000000000000200

French, D. (2024, January 14). Opinion | This is the actual danger posed by D.E.I. *New York Times* (nytimes.com). Accessed September 7, 2024.

Haggins, A. N. (2020). To be seen, heard, and valued: Strategies to promote a sense of belonging for women and underrepresented in medicine physicians. *Academic Medicine: Journal of the Association of American Medical Colleges*, 95(10), 1507–1510. https://doi.org/10.1097/ACM.0000000000003553

Helzer, E. G., Myers, C. G., Fahim, C., Sutcliffe, K. M., & Abernathy, J. H. (2020). Gender bias in collaborative medical decision making: Emergent evidence. *Academic Medicine: Journal of the Association of American Medical Colleges*, 95(10), 1524–1528. https://doi.org/10.1097/ACM.0000000000003590

Hoskison, K., & Beasley, B. W. (2019). A conversation about the role of humiliation in teaching: The ugly, the bad, and the good. *Academic Medicine: Journal of the Association of American Medical Colleges*, 94(8), 1078–1080. https://doi.org/10 .1097/ACM.0000000000002594

Lee, E. J., Ditchman, N., Thomas, J., & Tsen, J. (2019). Microaggressions experienced by people with multiple sclerosis in the workplace: An exploratory study using Sue's taxonomy. *Rehabilitation Psychology*, 64(2), 179–193. https://doi.org/10.1037/ rep0000269

Lockyer, J., de Groot, J., & Silver, I. (2016). Professional identity formation, the practicing physician and continuing professional development. In R. L. Cruess, S. R. Cruess, & Y. Steinert (Eds.), *Teaching medical professionalism: Supporting the development of a professional identity* (pp. 186–200). Cambridge University Press.

Manne-Goehler, J., Freund, K. M., Raj, A., Kaplan, S. E., Terrin, N., Breeze, J. L., & Carr, P. L. (2020). Evaluating the role of self-esteem on differential career outcomes by gender in academic medicine. *Academic Medicine: Journal of the Association of American Medical Colleges*, 95(10), 1558–1562. https://doi.org/10.1097/ACM .0000000000003138

Maristany, D., Hauer, K. E., Leep Hunderfund, A. N., Elks, M. L., Bullock, J. L., Kumbamu, A., & O'Brien, B. C. (2023). The problem and power of professionalism: A critical analysis of medical students' and residents' perspectives and experiences of professionalism. *Academic Medicine: Journal of the Association of American Medical Colleges*, 98(11S), S32–S41. https://doi.org/10.1097/ACM.0000000000005367

Molina, M. F., Landry, A. I., Chary, A. N., & Burnett-Bowie, S. M. (2020). Addressing the elephant in the room: Microaggressions in medicine. *Annals of Emergency Medicine*, 76(4), 387–391. https://doi.org/10.1016/j.annemergmed.2020.04.009

Pelley, E., & Carnes, M. (2020). When a specialty becomes "women's work": Trends in and implications of specialty gender segregation in medicine. *Academic Medicine: Journal of the Association of American Medical Colleges, 95*(10), 1499–1506. https://doi.org/10.1097/ACM.0000000000003555

Periyakoil, V. S., Chaudron, L., Hill, E. V., Pellegrini, V., Neri, E., & Kraemer, H. C. (2020). Common types of gender-based microaggressions in medicine. *Academic Medicine: Journal of the Association of American Medical Colleges, 95*(3), 450–457. https://doi.org/10.1097/ACM.0000000000003057

Reifler, D. R. (2015). The pedagogy of pimping: Educational rigor or mistreatment? *JAMA, 314*(22), 2355–2356. https://doi.org/10.1001/jama.2015.14670

Reifler, D. R. (2016). Pimping as a practice in medical education–Reply. *JAMA, 315*(20), 2237. https://doi.org/10.1001/jama.2016.1582

Reis, S. P. (2008). A horse of a different color. Personal communication.

Rogers, A. C., Wren, S. M., & McNamara, D. A. (2019). Gender and specialty influences on personal and professional life among trainees. *Annals of Surgery, 269*(2), 383–387. https://doi.org/10.1097/SLA.0000000000002580

Romanski, P. A., Bartz, D., Pelletier, A., & Johnson, N. R. (2020). The "invisible student": Neglect as a form of medical student mistreatment, a call to action. *Journal of Surgical Education, 77*(6), 1327–1330. https://doi.org/10.1016/j.jsurg.2020.05.013

Sharifi, M., Asadi-Pooya, A. A., & Mousavi-Roknabadi, R. S. (2020). Burnout among healthcare providers of COVID-19; A systematic review of epidemiology and recommendations. *Archives of Academic Emergency Medicine, 9*(1), e7. https://doi.org/10.22037/aaem.v9i1.1004

Simpson, D., Bidwell, J., La Fratta, T., & Agard, K. (2022). Using a milestone framework for assessing resident, fellow, and faculty competence in diversity, equity, and inclusion. *Journal of Graduate Medical Education, 14*(3), 342–343. https://doi.org/10.4300/JGME-D-21-00940.1

Stack, S. W., Eurich, K. E., Kaplan, E. A., Ball, A. L., Mookherjee, S., & Best, J. A. (2019). Parenthood during graduate medical education: A scoping review. *Academic Medicine: Journal of the Association of American Medical Colleges, 94*(11), 1814–1824. https://doi.org/10.1097/ACM.0000000000002948

Stack, S. W., Jagsi, R., Biermann, J. S., Lundberg, G. P., Law, K. L., Milne, C. K., Williams, S. G., Burton, T. C., Larison, C. L., & Best, J. A. (2020). Childbearing decisions in residency: A multicenter survey of female residents. *Academic Medicine: Journal of the Association of American Medical Colleges, 95*(10), 1550–1557. https://doi.org/10.1097/ACM.0000000000003549

Stack, S. W., McKinney, C. M., Spiekerman, C., & Best, J. A. (2018). Childbearing and maternity leave in residency: Determinants and well-being outcomes. *Postgraduate Medical Journal, 94*(1118), 694–699. https://doi.org/10.1136/postgradmedj-2018-135960

Sukhera, J., Kulkarni, C., & Taylor, T. (2021). Structural distress: Experiences of moral distress related to structural stigma during the COVID-19 pandemic. *Perspectives on Medical Education, 10*(4), 222–229. https://doi.org/10.1007/s40037-021-00663-y

Todd, A. R., Cawthorn, T. R., & Temple-Oberle, C. (2020). Pregnancy and parenthood remain challenging during surgical residency: A systematic review. *Academic Medicine: Journal of the Association of American Medical Colleges, 95*(10), 1607–1615. https://doi.org/10.1097/ACM.0000000000003351

Torres, M. B., Salles, A., & Cochran, A. (2019). Recognizing and reacting to microaggressions in medicine and surgery. *JAMA Surgery, 154*(9), 868–872. https://doi.org/10.1001/jamasurg.2019.1648

Trauma-Informed Care Toolkit | Center to Advance Palliative Care (capc.org).

Tyson, L., Skinner, J., Hariharan, B., Josiah, B., Okongwu, K., & Semlyen, J. (2024). Tackling discrimination in medicine head on: The impact of bystander intervention training. *Medical Teacher*, 1–10. Advance online publication. https://doi.org/10.1080/0142159X.2024.2316849

Wei, C., Bernstein, S. A., Gu, A., Mehta, A., Sharma, D., Mortman, R., Verduzco-Gutierrez, M., & Chretien, K. C. (2023). Evaluating diversity and inclusion content on graduate medical education websites. *Journal of General Internal Medicine*, *38*(3), 582–585. https://doi.org/10.1007/s11606-022-07973-9

Woodford, M. R., Howell, M. L., Kulick, A., & Silverschanz, P. (2013). "That's so gay": Heterosexual male undergraduates and the perpetuation of sexual orientation microaggressions on campus. *Journal of Interpersonal Violence*, *28*(2), 416–435. https://doi.org/10.1177/0886260512454719

Wyatt, T. R., Rockich-Winston, N., Taylor, T. R., & White, D. (2020). What does context have to do with anything? A study of professional identity formation in physician-trainees considered underrepresented in medicine. *Academic Medicine: Journal of the Association of American Medical Colleges*, *95*(10), 1587–1593. https://doi.org/10.1097/ACM.0000000000003192

Wyatt, T. R., Rockich-Winston, N., White, D., & Taylor, T. R. (2021). "Changing the narrative": A study on professional identity formation among Black/African American physicians in the U.S. *Advances in Health Sciences Education: Theory and Practice*, *26*(1), 183–198. https://doi.org/10.1007/s10459-020-09978-7

CHAPTER 8

The impact of COVID-19 on the doctor's life cycle

....

The redress of moral distress requires practical
wisdom, mutual trust, and supportive institutions

Emergency rooms in many parts of the country are seeing a dramatic rise in the number of patients seeking care. Beds are tight.

An experienced emergency room nurse describes the scene from the vantage point of the triage desk. He sits in full view of the large room of people worried enough to have sought ER care. Wearing a face mask and shield and ready with his stethoscope, a blood pressure cuff, thermometer, and oxygen monitor, he speaks with each arrival in turn, evaluating their situation and determining each person's level of urgency.

Coordinating with his colleagues who are treating patients behind the swinging double doors, he determines who will be seen next. Drawing on his well-developed sense of professionalism and years of clinical experience, he keeps track of the entire chaotic scene. The list reshuffles with each new arrival. Emotions are high. He interacts with those who question why people are not assigned ER beds in order of arrival and explains the triage process with empathy and patience.

Because of the pandemic, more and more people need urgent evaluation. There are not enough beds and staff. The triage nurse becomes even more vigilant as people are forced to wait longer and longer. He scans the waiting area, watching for subtle changes that might signal a COVID-19-related precipitous decline in respiratory stability. For each twelve-hour shift, he monitors the room and attends

DOI: 10.1201/9781003507529-9

to his other tasks. It is exhausting but rewarding. There is satisfaction in work done at the top of one's ability.

Then, one morning, an administrative leader comes by. The leader informs him of a new policy. Effective immediately, he will be required to document once an hour that each of the people in the waiting room is still safe. This will upend his routine. It will require a great deal of extra effort and take his attention away from monitoring the scene in front of him.

He knows that the institutional leader is asking him to document something that serves only to protect the institution from being accused of providing poor care. Instead of working to increase capacity, he realizes the institution is both avoiding its responsibilities and asking him to betray his values as a healthcare professional.

This situation, although not dramatic in the grand scheme of things, is a classic cause of moral distress.

"Moral distress" is a normal reaction to an abnormal situation. It is the psychological conflict that arises when "institutional constraints make it nearly impossible to pursue the right course of action,"[1] especially in high stakes moments. It has been described in health professionals, medical students, soldiers, social workers, police officers, teachers, and others. Although considered a normal response to abnormal and traumatic events, moral distress has also been associated with noxious mental and physical health consequences for healthcare workers including burnout, compassion fatigue, suicide, and permanently leaving the profession.

Since the beginning of the COVID-19 pandemic in 2020, healthcare workers around the world have dealt with surges in high acuity care and ethically challenging situations. In low- and middle-income countries, healthcare facilities were already stretched thin. In the US, reimbursement models have, for years, incentivized facilities to run at close-to-full capacity, leaving little slack to accommodate the pandemic.

As a result, the systemic stress has revealed how little we prepare and support our most precious resource, the people who make up the healthcare workforce. There was a nursing shortage *before* the pandemic. Studies of nurses and physicians conducted since the beginning of the COVID-19 pandemic show that 30–40% are seriously considering changing professions or retiring early. With each surge, more and more healthcare workers consider leaving.

So, how will we support the Class of 2025? The wellbeing of the professionals providing healthcare is related to the quality and safety of the care they provide, so we must help them develop strategies to weather the predictable and inherently demoralizing conflicts that can overwhelm their sense of goodness and humanity.

---

1   Mealer, M., & Moss, M. (2016). Moral distress in ICU nurses. *Intensive Care Medicine*, *42*(10), 1615–1617. https://doi.org/10.1007/s00134-016-4441-1

This past week, Dr. Catherine Ferguson told the brand-new Medical College of Wisconsin (MCW) medical students how we hope to prepare them to face down the inevitable challenges that accompany a career in medicine. Along with her colleagues, she has implemented an evidence-based, theory-informed REACH (Recognize, Empathize, Allow, Care, and Hold each other up)[2] curriculum to help them thrive by fostering knowledge, skills, relationships, and personal self-care habits.

The resilience which springs from a strength of character and clarity of conscience will push our students to "do the right thing at the right time for the right reasons," what Aristotle coined *practical wisdom*. Enhancing *individual* students' practical wisdom is not the entire answer, however. Patient quality and safety is a team sport, and we must also address systemic issues.

What is needed? To combat moral distress, we need to be able to trust each other and be trustworthy ourselves. Healthy work environments are characterized by reserves of trust, mutual respect, and caring that can be called to the forefront when the going gets tough. Creating a trustworthy healthcare environment takes time and attention aimed at intentionally building relationships and establishing shared values. Healthcare institutions that have made these investments can draw on them during crises. Healthcare systems have adapted during events like hurricanes and epidemics, but there is a long way to go.

The COVID-19 pandemic is not done with us and there are continuing challenges to our professions. Experts have proposed key strategies to address moral distress. These include enhanced decision-making support and more sharing of complex decision-making. For example, as in the story of the triage nurse, one clinician should not be left to make triage choices on their own. We must also provide adequate time and space for clinicians to decompress. Healthcare teams should be established and maintained in ways that enable trusting relationships to be nurtured. At the same time, institutional leadership and risk management professionals must listen intently to their frontline clinicians and staff, supporting changes in workflows that keep everyone safe, and reminding everyone of shared missions and goals.

At MCW, as is the case elsewhere around the country, our newest students will be caring for all of us well into the twenty-first century. This class has been selected from the largest pool of applicants ever to seek entry to medical and nursing schools, a phenomenon referred to as the "Fauci Effect" because of the

---

2   Ferguson, C. C., Ark, T. K., & Kalet, A. L. (2022). REACH: A required curriculum to foster the well-being of medical students. *Academic Medicine: Journal of the Association of American Medical Colleges*, 97(8), 1164–1169. https://doi.org/10.1097/ACM.0000000000004715

inspiration Anthony Fauci[3] provides with his stalwart, clear-eyed, scientifically rigorous and morally conscientious leadership. Paradoxically, these students are joining at a time when many clinicians are seriously considering leaving the profession.

This compels me to recommit to our mission of transforming medical education. Our students and colleagues must feel as though they are valued and cared for as they begin their journeys and be given the skills to thrive. Only then will we have given them the optimal opportunity to become superb, hardy healthcare professionals who strive to practice and care for others with compassion and practical wisdom.[4]

* * *

The opening story illustrates the tremendous clinical, moral, systemic, and existential challenges that the coronavirus pandemic engendered. It also encompasses and integrates many of the issues raised in former categories, from moral distress to character building, structural competence, practical wisdom, and the pervasive impact of external forces.

This category is emerging as essential, as the COVID-19 pandemic turned many practices and processes in healthcare and medical education upside down, mandating an urgent and comprehensive soul-searching concerning its impact on, among other areas, the present as well as future identity formation of physicians.[5]

Medicine and healthcare have been in fast and profound transition in recent decades,[6] with a further tectonic disruption by the pandemic. Among the many repercussions of these transitions, as stated in the Introduction, is that the doctor's life cycle (DLC) is already transforming as we are writing these lines. In more than one way, the analysis in the relevant literature of the pandemic's impact on healthcare systems,

---

3* Anthony S. Fauci, MD, is an American physician-scientist and immunologist who served as the Director of the National Institute of Allergy and Infectious Diseases from 1984 to 2022. He was the Chief Medical Advisor to the President of the United States from 2021 to 2022 during the worst days of the COVID-19 pandemic, appearing on national television nightly for most of that time.

4 Kalet, A. (2021, August 13). The redress of moral distress requires practical wisdom, mutual trust and supportive institutions. *Transformational Times: Newsletter of the Robert D. and Patricia E. Kern Institute for the Transformation of Medical Education.*

5 Keesara, S., Jonas, A., & Schulman, K. (2020). Covid-19 and health care's digital revolution. *New England Journal of Medicine, 382*(23), e82. https://doi.org/10.1056/NEJMp2005835

6 Narayan, K. M. V., Curran, J. W., & Foege, W. H. (2021). The COVID-19 pandemic as an opportunity to ensure a more successful future for science and public health. *JAMA, 325*(6), 525–526. https://doi.org/10.1001/jama.2020.23479

health professions education,[7,8,9,10,11,12,13,14,15,16] and professional identity formation (PIF), as well as the ensuing recommendations, validate former categories while signaling that the forecasted transitions are now augmented by various factors. These include the pandemic disruptions, predicted significant technological and scientific advances, climate change, racism, political polarization, and wars. These transitions, disruptions, and transformations, from micro to macro levels, clearly impact the present and future of healthcare systems and outcomes, as well as the DLC.

7   Montagna, E., Donohoe, J., Zaia, V., Duggan, E., O'Leary, P., Waddington, J., & O'Tuathaigh, C. (2021). Transition to clinical practice during the COVID-19 pandemic: A qualitative study of young doctors' experiences in Brazil and Ireland. *BMJ Open, 11*(9), e053423. https://doi.org/10.1136/bmjopen-2021-053423

8   Gordon, M., Patricio, M., Horne, L., Muston, A., Alston, S. R., Pammi, M., Thammasitboon, S., Park, S., Pawlikowska, T., Rees, E. L., Doyle, A. J., & Daniel, M. (2020). Developments in medical education in response to the COVID-19 pandemic: A rapid BEME systematic review: BEME Guide No. 63. *Medical Teacher, 42*(11), 1202–1215. https://doi.org/10.1080/0142159X.2020.1807484

9   Govender, L., & de Villiers, M. R. (2021). When disruption strikes the curriculum: Towards a crisis-curriculum analysis framework. *Medical Teacher, 43*(6), 694–699. https://doi.org/10.1080/0142159X.2021.1887839

10 Southworth, E., & Gleason, S. H. (2021). COVID 19: A cause for pause in undergraduate medical education and catalyst for innovation. *HEC Forum: An Interdisciplinary Journal on Hospitals' Ethical and Legal Issues, 33*(1–2), 125–142. https://doi.org/10.1007/s10730-020-09433-5

11 Byram, J. N., Frankel, R. M., Isaacson, J. H., & Mehta, N. (2022). The impact of COVID-19 on professional identity. *Clinical Teacher, 19*(3), 205–212. https://doi.org/10.1111/tct.13467

12 Findyartini, A., Anggraeni, D., Husin, J. M., & Greviana, N. (2020). Exploring medical students' professional identity formation through written reflections during the COVID-19 pandemic. *Journal of Public Health Research, 9*(Suppl 1), 1918. https://doi.org/10.4081/jphr.2020.1918

13 Harvey, A. B., Brown, M., Byrne, M., Alexander, L., Wan, J., Ashcroft, J., Schindler, N., & Brassett, C. (2021). "I don't feel like I'm learning to be a doctor": Early insights regarding the impact of Covid-19 on UK medical student professional identity. *medRxiv, 8*. https://doi.org/10.1101/2021.08.01.21261101

14 Muller, D., Parkas, V., Amiel, J., Anand, S., Cassese, T., Cunningham, T., Kang, Y., Nosanchuk, J., Soriano, R., Zbar, L., & Karani, R. (2021). Guiding principles for undergraduate medical education in the time of the COVID-19 pandemic. *Medical Teacher, 43*(2), 137–141. https://doi.org/10.1080/0142159X.2020.1841892

15 Humphrey, H. J., Sharp-McHenry, L., & Whelan, A. J. (2022). Pandemic exposes imperative to transform health professions education. *Academic Medicine: Journal of the Association of American Medical Colleges, 97*(3S), S1–S2. https://doi.org/10.1097/ACM.0000000000004505

16 Triemstra, J. D., Haas, M. R. C., Bhavsar-Burke, I., Gottlieb-Smith, R., Wolff, M., Shelgikar, A. V., Samala, R. V., Ruff, A. L., Kuo, K., Tam, M., Gupta, A., Stojan, J., Gruppen, L., & Ellinas, H. (2021). Impact of the COVID-19 pandemic on the clinical learning environment: Addressing identified gaps and seizing opportunities. *Academic Medicine: Journal of the Association of American Medical Colleges, 96*(9), 1276–1281. https://doi.org/10.1097/ACM.0000000000004013

Indeed, in this brave new world, transformative learning is promoted as a goal for the individual health professional and adaptation to radical change is imperative. Also, the deficiencies and shortcomings of global and national healthcare systems uncovered by the pandemic, along with the accompanying challenges, necessitate a major shift in how healthcare is conceptualized and delivered. In addition, immense ethical and humane challenges created by the pandemic were brought to the fore[17,18,19,20,21,22] in tandem with the impact of unprecedented current and anticipated technological progress.[23] In particular, the pandemic highlighted the ubiquity of moral distress and injury experienced by health professionals and the profound negative impact it had on their wellbeing (see Chapter 4 and the opening narrative of this chapter).

THE IMPACT OF COVID-19 ON HEALTHCARE AND PUBLIC HEALTH

The pandemic exposed the severe limitations of healthcare systems, especially with respect to health equity and the impact of digital

17 Montauk, T. R., & Kuhl, E. A. (2020). COVID-related family separation and trauma in the intensive care unit. *Psychological Trauma: Theory, Research, Practice and Policy, 12*(S1), S96–S97. https://doi.org/10.1037/tra0000839

18 Sarkar, U., & Cassel, C. (2021). Humanism before heroism in medicine. *JAMA, 326*(2), 127–128. https://doi.org/10.1001/jama.2021.9569

19 Skochelak, S. E., Lomis, K. D., Andrews, J. S., Hammoud, M. M., Mejicano, G. C., & Byerley, J. (2021). Realizing the vision of the Lancet Commission on education of health professionals for the 21st century: Transforming medical education through the accelerating change in medical education consortium. *Medical Teacher, 43*(Suppl 2), S1–S6. https://doi.org/10.1080/0142159X.2021.1935833

20 Hughes, M. T., & Rushton, C. H. (2022). Ethics and well-being: The health professions and the COVID-19 pandemic. *Academic Medicine: Journal of the Association of American Medical Colleges, 97*(3S), S98–S103. https://doi.org/10.1097/ACM.0000000000004524

21 Cherak, S. J., Brown, A., Kachra, R., Makuk, K., Sudershan, S., Paget, M., & Kassam, A. (2021). Exploring the impact of the COVID-19 pandemic on medical learner wellness: A needs assessment for the development of learner wellness interventions. *Canadian Medical Education Journal, 12*(3), 54–69. https://doi.org/10.36834/cmej.70995

22 Farrell, C. M., & Hayward, B. J. (2022). Ethical dilemmas, moral distress, and the risk of moral injury: Experiences of residents and fellows during the COVID-19 pandemic in the United States. *Academic Medicine: Journal of the Association of American Medical Colleges, 97*(3S), S55–S60. https://doi.org/10.1097/ACM.0000000000004536

23 Barach, P., Fisher, S. D., Adams, M. J., Burstein, G. R., Brophy, P. D., Kuo, D. Z., & Lipshultz, S. E. (2020). Disruption of healthcare: Will the COVID pandemic worsen non-COVID outcomes and disease outbreaks? *Progress in Pediatric Cardiology, 59*, 101254. https://doi.org/10.1016/j.ppedcard.2020.101254

technology (Kuhlmann).[24] The disproportionately high rate of morbidity and premature death among economically and socially marginalized populations was profound. Women, whether health professionals or part of the general population, shouldered an extra burden in their homes.[25] In the United States, "COVID-19 has disrupted every aspect of the U.S. health care and health professions education systems, creating anxiety, suffering, and chaos and exposing many of the flaws in the nation's public health, medical education, and political systems."[26] Many believe that this awakened Americans "to the limitations of their analogue health care system," making it clear that "an immediate digital revolution to face this crisis" was needed. Furthermore:

> The U.S. health care industry is structured on the historically necessary model of in-person interactions between patients and their clinicians. Clinical workflows and economic incentives have largely been developed to support and reinforce a face-to-face model of care, resulting in the congregation of patients in emergency departments and waiting areas during this crisis.

One forward-thinking perspective for healthcare in the United States is that "models of care that have been dominant in the past will likely give way to new approaches to providing health care that come with new workforce needs."[27] The pandemic forced a dual view: first, its macrolevel impact on systems, illustrating the profound impact of external forces, and second, its impact on the micro-level reality of the clinical encounter, raising doubts about a multitude of sacred cows.

THE IMPACT OF COVID-19 ON DOCTORING

In primary care, there was a complete reversal in the point of care with a disruptive and confusing message: *If you are sick, stay home, don't*

24 Kuhlmann, E., Dussault, G., & Correia, T. (2021). Global health and health workforce development: What to learn from COVID-19 on health workforce preparedness and resilience. *The International Journal of Health Planning and Management*, 36(S1), 5–8. https://doi.org/10.1002/hpm.3160

25 Roberts, L. W. (2020). Women and academic medicine, 2020. *Academic Medicine: Journal of the Association of American Medical Colleges*, 95(10), 1459–1464. https://doi.org/10.1097/ACM.0000000000003617

26 Sklar, D.P. (2020). COVID-19: Lessons from the disaster that can improve health professions education. *Academic Medicine*, 95(11), 1631-3. https://doi.org/10.1097/ACM.0000000000003547

27 Wilensky, G. R. (2022, January 4). The COVID-19 pandemic and the US health care workforce. *JAMA Health Forum*, 3(1), e220001. American Medical Association.

come to see me.[28] Practitioners became fearful of their patients, lest they infect them. Personal protective equipment added another surreal and disruptive dimension. The profound ethical challenge of the duty of care versus the duty to attend to the healer's risk on the job became pervasive. Health professionals, including learners, contracted COVID-19, often on the job, and some succumbed to it. Dying in the ICU, under necessary protective isolation, with no loved ones by the dying patient's side, and with care providers avoiding human touch, created moral and emotional distress.

In the face of this catastrophe, dedication, altruism, and resilience also emerged, drawing appreciation and gratitude from patients, families, and communities. After the initial shock, healthcare teams experienced pride in their essential and selfless contributions, often in contrast with former tenuous, conflictual, and untrusting experiences. Still, as **Hughes** and **Rushton** state:

> The COVID-19 pandemic has had a profound impact on health professionals, adding to the moral suffering and burnout that existed prepandemic. The physical, psychological, and moral toll of the pandemic has threatened the well-being and integrity of clinicians. The narrative of self-sacrifice and heroism bolstered people early on but was not sustainable over time.[29]

Further, they assert that "investing in the well-being and resilience of clinicians, implementing the recommendations of the National Academy of Medicine, and engaging learners and faculty as cocreators of ethical practice have the potential to transform the learning environment."

The pandemic also transformed learners' and practitioners' landscape of moral concerns. **Farrell** and **Hayward**[30] describe their experiences working in pulmonary and critical care in New York City during

28 Lin, S., Sattler, A., & Smith, M. (2020). Retooling primary care in the COVID-19 era. *Mayo Clinic Proceedings, 95*(9), 1831–1834. https://doi.org/10.1016/j.mayocp.2020.06.050

29 Hughes, M. T., & Rushton, C. H. (2022). Ethics and well-being: The health professions and the COVID-19 pandemic. Academic Medicine: *Journal of the Association of American Medical Colleges, 97*(3S), S98–S103. https://doi.org/10.1097/ACM.0000000000004524

30 Farrell, C. M., & Hayward, B. J. (2022). Ethical dilemmas, moral distress, and the risk of moral injury: Experiences of residents and fellows during the COVID-19 pandemic in the United States. Academic Medicine: *Journal of the Association of American Medical Colleges, 97*(3S), S55–S60. https://doi.org/10.1097/ACM.0000000000004536

the pandemic, supplemented by the literature, as follows: "Common ethical dilemmas confronted by residents and fellows during the pandemic … are related to personal health risk, resource allocation, health care inequities, and media relations." They underline how the combined stress of training and the pandemic increased the potential for trainee moral distress and the ensuing "risk for moral injury with consequences for their mental health and overall well-being."

THE IMPACT OF COVID-19 ON MEDICAL EDUCATION

Medical education was initially suspended, then preclinical studies were transferred to a virtual environment with clinical education in limbo. Residents were redeployed as care needs prevailed, often away from their discipline of choice. As Hughes and Rushton describe:

> For health professions students, the learning environment changed dramatically, limiting opportunities in direct patient care and raising concerns for meeting training requirements. Learners lost social connections and felt isolated while learning remotely, and they witnessed ethical tensions between patient-centered care and parallel obligations to public health. Worries about transmission of the virus and uncertainty about its management contributed to their moral suffering. Educators adjusted curricula to address the changing ethical landscape.[31]

A systematic review identified that "the focus of developments included pivoting to online learning (n = 58), simulation (n = 24), assessment (n = 11), well-being (n = 8), telehealth (n = 5), clinical service reconfigurations (n = 4), interviews (n = 4), service provision (n = 2), faculty development (n = 2) and other (n = 9)."[32] A major disruption concerned teaching clinical skills, which transitioned from "bedside" to "web-side and lab-side."[33] However, this shift was deemed acceptable by many students

31 Hughes, M. T., & Rushton, C. H. (2022). Ethics and well-being: The health professions and the COVID-19 pandemic. Academic Medicine: *Journal of the Association of American Medical Colleges*, 97(3S), S98–S103. https://doi.org/10.1097/ACM.0000000000004524

32 Daniel, M., Gordon, M., Patricio, M., Hider, A., Pawlik, C., Bhagdev, R., Ahmad, S., Alston, S., Park, S., Pawlikowska, T., & Rees, E. (2021, March 4). An update on developments in medical education in response to the COVID-19 pandemic: A BEME scoping review: BEME Guide No. 64. *Medical Teacher*, 43(3), 253–271.

33 Tsang, A. C. O., Shih, K. C., & Chen, J. Y. (2021). Clinical skills education at the bed-side, web-side and lab-side. *Medical Education*, 55(1), 112–114. https://doi.org/10.1111/medu.14394

and signifies that "on the learner side, self-directed learning may become more important as learners will need to navigate the multitude of materials available online."

Constrained by COVID-19 restrictions, educators introduced educational interventions and curricular changes with a marked increase in web-based educational experiences and simulation in lieu of patient contact, as well as coaching, reflective writing, service learning (offering students direct patient care opportunities beyond their developmental stage), or discipline (for residents)—sometimes also called experience-based medical education.[34,35] The pandemic also demonstrated how an urgent disruption mandates a new educational priority and leaves a legacy that disaster medicine (pandemics, natural disasters, armed conflicts, and so on) should move from the periphery of curricula to a more central position. A key role was identified for palliative care, along with several marginalized and often absent clinical domains—namely, end-of-life care, disaster medicine, bioethics, and physician and learner wellbeing—that became central and of top curricular priority during the pandemic.[36]

Southworth and **Gleason**[37] are concerned with the hidden curriculum: "The implicit way in which social and cultural aspects of an environment impart knowledge and mold behavior—known as the hidden curriculum—is especially pervasive in the house of medicine and can be the most powerful teacher in times of uncertainty." They qualify the pandemic as "one of the purest experiments in medical education's hidden curriculum: students are navigating a system without much explanation or guidance as practice and policy change almost daily."

They raise the following issues:

---

34 Dixon, W., Gallegos, M., & Williams, S. (2022). A brief coaching pilot enhances professional identity formation and clinical skills acquisition during emergency medicine clerkships shortened by COVID-19. *Western Journal of Emergency Medicine*, 23(1), 30–32. https://doi.org/10.5811/westjem.2021.12.53917

35 Costello, M., Cantillon, P., Geoghegan, R., Byrne, D., Lowery, A., & Walsh, S. M. (2022). Experience-based learning: How a crisis solution informed fundamental change in a clinical education curriculum. *Clinical Teacher*, 19(1), 42–47. https://doi.org/10.1111/tct.13441

36 Radbruch, L., Knaul, F. M., de Lima, L., de Joncheere, C., & Bhadelia, A. (2020). The key role of palliative care in response to the COVID-19 tsunami of suffering. *Lancet*, 395(10235), 1467–1469. https://doi.org/10.1016/S0140-6736(20)30964-8

37 Southworth, E., & Gleason, S. H. (2021). COVID 19: A cause for pause in undergraduate medical education and catalyst for innovation. HEC Forum: *An Interdisciplinary Journal on Hospitals' Ethical and Legal Issues*, 33(1–2), 125–142. https://doi.org/10.1007/s10730-020-09433-5

The actions taken during this time signal to students what is important, who is important, and how to adapt during a global crisis. Sudden and dramatic changes to time-honored curricula, testing, and interview processes make us question how essential these traditions truly are to undergraduate medical education. … Should we return to the pre-pandemic ways of educating, assessing, and recruiting? Will students ever return to face-to-face didactics? Perhaps not, and maybe this makes way for innovations.

Further, they also ask:

If COVID-19's legacy is a toxic hidden curriculum, then we might expect worsening of current discouraging trends in medical training and practice. For example, … will it exacerbate empathy erosion or will it perhaps broaden trainees' understanding of population-based medicine, translational research, and utilitarian principles of healthcare ethics? Will students feel disenfranchised or will they speak up about their educational and professional fates as they did when confronted with sudden changes to USMLE [United States Medical Licensing Examination] test-taking procedures?

And:

"COVID-19 compels us to examine the utility and ethics of undergraduate medical educational practices that may benefit a majority but leave a portion of students disadvantaged. What lasting impact will COVID-19 have on the current cohort of trainees?"

THE IMPACT OF COVID-19 ON PROFESSIONAL IDENTITY FORMATION

As already stated, the disruptive impact of the pandemic did not spare PIF. As this impact is still largely unknown, some of the related literature is somewhat speculative.[38,39]

---

38 Rehman, M., Khalid, F., Sheth, U., Al-Duaij, L., Chow, J., Azim, A., Last, N., Blissett, S., & Sibbald, M. (2024). Quarantining from professional identity: How did COVID-19 impact professional identity formation in undergraduate medical education? *Perspectives on Medical Education, 13*(1), 130–140. https://doi.org/10.5334/pme.1308

39 Cupido, N., Diamond, L., Kulasegaram, K., Martimianakis, M. A., & Forte, M. (2023). Detour or new direction: The impact of the COVID-19 pandemic on the professional identity formation of postgraduate residents. *Academic Medicine: Journal of the Association of American Medical Colleges, 98*(11S), S24–S31. https://doi.org/10.1097/ACM.0000000000005359

Scholars predict that emerging physician identities will be inter-professional rather than intraprofessional[40] as a result of exposure to the vital importance of teamwork, volunteers, and collaboration across multiple professions during the pandemic, which sent a "strong message that learning about, from, and with other professions is critically important."[41] A need has been identified for diversifying PIF in nontraditional ways, such as by placing learners in public health roles, increasing service learning, or supervising social media.

Furthermore, attention is being called to the increased identity work required to reconcile one's racial, gender, and other identities with that of the physician. As conveyed by a female Black resident: "I have not mastered the art of reconciling my identity as a Black woman with my identity as a physician. I frequently feel I have to silence the Black woman and simply be a physician, colorless, un-Black."[42] This profoundly connects the former category to the current one. **Stetson** and **Dhaliwal** quote **Frost** and **Regehr**, who advocate the goal "that all students are able to construct identities as physicians that will allow them to retain and take advantage of their individuality while respecting and honoring professional values and norms."[43] Nevertheless, "the boundary conditions for professionalism will continue to shift, and with that will come a necessary evolution in PIF instructional methods and activities." An adaptation illustrative of this change was presented by **Huddart** et al., who reported how a United Kingdom-based national organization used a Twitter (now X) chat to coordinate medical student COVID-19-related volunteering efforts, including nonclinical work like grocery shopping and combating misinformation.[44] The group's name was "Becoming a Doctor."

40 Stetson, G. V., & Dhaliwal, G. (2021). Using a time out: Reimagining professional identity formation after the pandemic. *Medical Education, 55*(1), 131–134. https://doi.org/10.1111/medu.14386

41 Kent, F., George, J., Lindley, J., & Brock, T. (2020). Virtual workshops to preserve interprofessional collaboration when physical distancing. *Medical Education, 54,* 661–662. https://doi.org/10.1111/medu.14179

42 AbdelHameid, D. (2020, July 30). Professionalism 101 for Black physicians. *New England Journal of Medicine, 383*(5), e34.

43 Stetson, G. V., & Dhaliwal, G. (2021). Using a time out: Reimagining professional identity formation after the pandemic. *Medical Education, 55*(1), 131–134. https://doi.org/10.1111/medu.14386

44 Huddart, D., Hirniak, J., Sethi, R., Hayer, G., Dibblin, C., Meghna Rao, B., Ehsaanuz Zaman, M., Jenkins, C., Hueso, B., & Sethi, S. (2020). #MedStudentCovid: How social media is supporting students during COVID-19. *Medical Education, 54*(10), 951–952. https://doi.org/10.1111/medu.14215

Reviewing the impact of COVID-19 on PIF, Stetson and Dhaliwal have come up with five pull-out points:

[1]   Observers wondered if preserving or advancing students' professional identity and professionalism while away from patients and colleagues was possible. …

[2]   Academic credit for COVID-19-related service is a first step in signalling to students that these skills and activities are a must-have. …

[3]   Educators designed integrated approaches to volunteer and education efforts that emphasised collaboration across professions during the crisis. …

[4]   Treat social media skills as a professional competency rather than a professional landmine. …

[5]   The pandemic-induced pause on training provided an opportunity to envision a more community focused, interprofessional, interconnected and inclusive conceptualisation of professional identity formation.

SCHOLAR RECOMMENDATIONS FOR ADDRESSING CONCERNS RAISED BY COVID-19

Scholar recommendations span several themes. First is disparities and how they are addressed in healthcare and education. As **Kinnear** et al. suggest:

> By taking this moment of crisis to examine the values and norms of medicine and how we systematically perpetuate harmful inequities and biases, we have an opportunity to deliberately rebuild our community of practice in a manner that helps shape the next generation's professional identities to be better than we have been. This should always be the aim of education.[45]

A second theme addresses medical, moral, and PIF education innovation. Hughes and Rushton recommend: "Preparing learners for the realities of their future professional identities requires creation of interprofessional moral communities that provide support and help develop the moral agency and integrity of its members using experiential and relational learning methods."[46] They add:

45   Kinnear, B., Zhou, C., Kinnear, B., Carraccio, C., & Schumacher, D. J. (2021). Professional identity formation during the COVID-19 pandemic. *Journal of Hospital Medicine, 16*(1), 44–46. https://doi.org/10.12788/jhm.3540

46   Hughes, M. T., & Rushton, C. H. (2022). Ethics and well-being: The health professions and the COVID-19 pandemic. *Academic Medicine: Journal of the Association of American Medical Colleges, 97*(3S), S98–S103. https://doi.org/10.1097/ACM.0000000000004524

Faculty need to be trained as effective mentors to create safe spaces for exploring challenges and address moral adversity. Ethics education will need to expand to issues related to health systems science, social determinants of health, and public health, and the cultivation of moral sensitivity, character development, professional identity formation, and moral resilience.

Lucey et al. summarize their overall recommendations for transforming medical education, casting them into a concrete plan (Table 8.1):

We have no choice but to transform. ... The authors suggest that medical education is at such an inflection point and propose a transformational vision of the medical education ecosystem, followed by a 10-year, 10-point plan that focuses on building the workforce that will achieve that vision. Broad themes include adopting a national vision; enhancing medicine's role in social justice through broadened curricula and a focus on communities; establishing equity in learning and processes related to learning, including wellness in learners, as a baseline; and realizing the promise of competency-based, time-variable training.[47]

The pandemic touched upon all facets of healthcare and medical education. Hopefully, as the coronavirus declines worldwide, its impact on the becoming and being of the physician will continue to become clearer. Meanwhile, the cited recommendations may be the best course of action for a benevolent transformation of healthcare and doctoring, medical education, and PIF.

For the first five categories analyzed in this book, the literature is many decades old and the findings robust and stable. For the three subsequent categories—the wounded healer and remediation (category 6); bias, gender, and race (category 7); and constructs highlighted in this category such as moral distress and injury—the literature is profoundly impacted by both the pandemic (an urgent, massive, and disruptive natural event) and coincident powerful societal, political, economic, and technological shifts. We assert that these are the three domains of the DLC discourse where scholarly attention is most urgent.

---

47 Lucey, C. R., Davis, J. A., & Green, M. M. (2022). We have no choice but to transform: The future of medical education after the COVID-19 pandemic. *Academic Medicine: Journal of the Association of American Medical Colleges*, 97(3S), S71–S81. https://doi.org/10.1097/ACM.0000000000004526

TABLE 8.1 A 10-Point, 10-Year Platform for Medical Education Transformation

1. Adopt a national vision of the successful workforce focused on committing to improving health and health care in all communities across the country.
2. Achieve social justice in medical education and health care across the country by actively seeking out and eliminating the consequences and manifestations of structural racism in medicine and medical education.
3. Design curricula to prepare all in the physician workforce, present and future, to embrace the breadth of roles and responsibilities needed to address syndemic causes of suffering from illness and disease.
4. Identify and address the most pressing causes of morbidity and mortality in communities across the nation by challenging medical education programs to partner with local communities and governments to focus educational programs on these issues.
5. Facilitate growth mindsets and support lifelong learning in future physicians—and promote equity in learning environments—by adopting a standard of programmatic assessment strategies across the continuum of medical education.
6. Protect patient safety while improving efficiency of training by implementing competency-based training.
7. Increase equity, affordability, effectiveness, and efficiency of selection processes by redesigning national systems and investing in national technology platforms.
8. Protect the workforce by prioritizing learner and physician well-being.
9. Address health care access issues for underserved communities across the nation through innovative partnerships.
10. Strengthen and promulgate the social contract between the medical profession, the public, and state and federal governments in support of health and well-being.

Source: Reproduced with permission from Wolters Kluwer Health, Inc.

Summary

As the global community is hopefully recovering from the impact of the COVID-19 pandemic, the shock waves are very much still felt in healthcare and medical education. There is no telling yet how this shared experience has impacted the DLC or how it will change it in the future. However, based on parallel historical events such as the influenza, tuberculosis, and HIV pandemics, as well as social upheavals and conflicts including wars and natural disasters, significant disruption of the DLC can be expected. Since embarking on this project, we have come to understand that the DLC terrain is not nearly as well charted as we had once believed. Where do we go from here?

REFERENCES

AbdelHameid, D. (2020, July 30). Professionalism 101 for Black physicians. *New England Journal of Medicine*, 383(5), e34.

Barach, P., Fisher, S. D., Adams, M. J., Burstein, G. R., Brophy, P. D., Kuo, D. Z., & Lipshultz, S. E. (2020). Disruption of healthcare: Will the COVID pandemic worsen non-COVID outcomes and disease outbreaks? *Progress in Pediatric Cardiology*, 59, 101254. https://doi.org/10.1016/j.ppedcard.2020.101254

Byram, J. N., Frankel, R. M., Isaacson, J. H., & Mehta, N. (2022). The impact of COVID-19 on professional identity. *Clinical Teacher*, 19(3), 205–212. https://doi.org/10.1111/tct.13467

Cherak, S. J., Brown, A., Kachra, R., Makuk, K., Sudershan, S., Paget, M., & Kassam, A. (2021). Exploring the impact of the COVID-19 pandemic on medical learner wellness: A needs assessment for the development of learner wellness interventions. *Canadian Medical Education Journal*, 12(3), 54–69. https://doi.org/10.36834/cmej.70995

Costello, M., Cantillon, P., Geoghegan, R., Byrne, D., Lowery, A., & Walsh, S. M. (2022). Experience-based learning: How a crisis solution informed fundamental change in a clinical education curriculum. *Clinical Teacher*, 19(1), 42–47. https://doi.org/10.1111/tct.13441

Cupido, N., Diamond, L., Kulasegaram, K., Martimianakis, M. A., & Forte, M. (2023). Detour or new direction: The impact of the COVID-19 pandemic on the professional identity formation of postgraduate residents. *Academic Medicine: Journal of the Association of American Medical Colleges*, 98(11S), S24–S31. https://doi.org/10.1097/ACM.0000000000005359

Daniel, M., Gordon, M., Patricio, M., Hider, A., Pawlik, C., Bhagdev, R., Ahmad, S., Alston, S,. Park, S., Pawlikowska, T., & Rees, E. (2021, March 4). An update on developments in medical education in response to the COVID-19 pandemic: A BEME scoping review: BEME Guide No. 64. *Medical Teacher*, 43(3), 253–271.

Dixon, W., Gallegos, M., & Williams, S. (2022). A brief coaching pilot enhances professional identity formation and clinical skills acquisition during emergency medicine clerkships shortened by COVID-19. *Western Journal of Emergency Medicine*, 23(1), 30–32. https://doi.org/10.5811/westjem.2021.12.53917

Farrell, C. M., & Hayward, B. J. (2022). Ethical dilemmas, moral distress, and the risk of moral injury: Experiences of residents and fellows during the COVID-19 pandemic in the United States. *Academic Medicine: Journal of the Association of American Medical Colleges*, 97(3S), S55–S60. https://doi.org/10.1097/ACM.0000000000004536

Ferguson, C. C., Ark, T. K., & Kalet, A. L. (2022). REACH: A required curriculum to foster the well-being of medical students. *Academic Medicine: Journal of the Association of American Medical Colleges*, 97(8), 1164–1169. https://doi.org/10.1097/ACM.0000000000004715

Findyartini, A., Anggraeni, D., Husin, J. M., & Greviana, N. (2020). Exploring medical students' professional identity formation through written reflections during the COVID-19 pandemic. *Journal of Public Health Research*, 9(Suppl 1), 1918. https://doi.org/10.4081/jphr.2020.1918

Gordon, M., Patricio, M., Horne, L., Muston, A., Alston, S. R., Pammi, M., Thammasitboon, S., Park, S., Pawlikowska, T., Rees, E. L., Doyle, A. J., & Daniel, M. (2020). Developments in medical education in response to the COVID-19 pandemic: A rapid BEME systematic review: BEME Guide No. 63. *Medical Teacher*, 42(11), 1202–1215. https://doi.org/10.1080/0142159X.2020.1807484

Govender, L., & de Villiers, M. R. (2021). When disruption strikes the curriculum: Towards a crisis-curriculum analysis framework. *Medical Teacher*, 43(6), 694–699. https://doi.org/10.1080/0142159X.2021.1887839

Harvey, A. B, Brown, M., Byrne, M., Alexander, L., Wan, J., Ashcroft, J., Schindler, N., & Brassett, C. (2021). "I don't feel like I'm learning to be a doctor": Early insights regarding the impact of Covid-19 on UK medical student professional identity. *medRxiv*, 8. https://doi.org/10.1101/2021.08.01.21261101

Huddart, D., Hirniak, J., Sethi, R., Hayer, G., Dibblin, C., Meghna Rao, B., Ehsaanuz Zaman, M., Jenkins, C., Hueso, B., & Sethi, S. (2020). #MedStudentCovid: How social media is supporting students during COVID-19. *Medical Education*, *54*(10), 951–952. https://doi.org/10.1111/medu.14215

Hughes, M. T., & Rushton, C. H. (2022). Ethics and well-being: The health professions and the COVID-19 pandemic. *Academic Medicine: Journal of the Association of American Medical Colleges*, *97*(3S), S98–S103. https://doi.org/10.1097/ACM.0000000000004524

Humphrey, H. J., Sharp-McHenry, L., & Whelan, A. J. (2022). Pandemic exposes imperative to transform health professions education. *Academic Medicine: Journal of the Association of American Medical Colleges*, *97*(3S), S1–S2. https://doi.org/10.1097/ACM.0000000000004505

Kalet, A. (2021, August 13). The redress of moral distress requires practical wisdom, mutual trust, and supportive institutions. *Transformational Times: Newsletter of the Robert D. and Patricia E. Kern Institute for the Transformation of Medical Education*.

Keesara, S., Jonas, A., & Schulman, K. (2020). Covid-19 and health care's digital revolution. *New England Journal of Medicine*, *382*(23), e82. https://doi.org/10.1056/NEJMp2005835

Kent, F., George, J., Lindley, J., & Brock, T. (2020). Virtual workshops to preserve interprofessional collaboration when physical distancing. *Medical Education*, *54*, 661–662. https://doi.org/10.1111/medu.14179

Kinnear, B., Zhou, C., Kinnear, B., Carraccio, C., & Schumacher, D. J. (2021). Professional identity formation during the COVID-19 pandemic. *Journal of Hospital Medicine*, *16*(1), 44–46. https://doi.org/10.12788/jhm.3540

Kuhlmann, E., Dussault, G., & Correia, T. (2021). Global health and health workforce development: What to learn from COVID-19 on health workforce preparedness and resilience. *International Journal of Health Planning and Management*, *36*(S1), 5–8. https://doi.org/10.1002/hpm.3160

Lin, S., Sattler, A., & Smith, M. (2020). Retooling primary care in the COVID-19 era. *Mayo Clinic Proceedings*, *95*(9), 1831–1834. https://doi.org/10.1016/j.mayocp.2020.06.050

Lucey, C. R., Davis, J. A., & Green, M. M. (2022). We have no choice but to transform: The future of medical education after the COVID-19 pandemic. *Academic Medicine: Journal of the Association of American Medical Colleges*, *97*(3S), S71–S81. https://doi.org/10.1097/ACM.0000000000004526

Mealer, M., & Moss, M. (2016). Moral distress in ICU nurses. *Intensive Care Medicine*, *42*(10), 1615–1617. https://doi.org/10.1007/s00134-016-4441-1

Montagna, E., Donohoe, J., Zaia, V., Duggan, E., O'Leary, P., Waddington, J., & O'Tuathaigh, C. (2021). Transition to clinical practice during the COVID-19 pandemic: A qualitative study of young doctors' experiences in Brazil and Ireland. *BMJ Open*, *11*(9), e053423. https://doi.org/10.1136/bmjopen-2021-053423

Montauk, T. R., & Kuhl, E. A. (2020). COVID-related family separation and trauma in the intensive care unit. *Psychological Trauma: Theory, Research, Practice and Policy*, *12*(S1), S96–S97. https://doi.org/10.1037/tra0000839

Muller, D., Parkas, V., Amiel, J., Anand, S., Cassese, T., Cunningham, T., Kang, Y., Nosanchuk, J., Soriano, R., Zbar, L., & Karani, R. (2021). Guiding principles for undergraduate medical education in the time of the COVID-19 pandemic. *Medical Teacher*, *43*(2), 137–141. https://doi.org/10.1080/0142159X.2020.1841892

Narayan, K. M. V., Curran, J. W., & Foege, W. H. (2021). The COVID-19 pandemic as an opportunity to ensure a more successful future for science and public health. *JAMA*, *325*(6), 525–526. https://doi.org/10.1001/jama.2020.23479

Radbruch, L., Knaul, F. M., de Lima, L., de Joncheere, C., & Bhadelia, A. (2020). The key role of palliative care in response to the COVID-19 tsunami of suffering. *Lancet*, *395*(10235), 1467–1469. https://doi.org/10.1016/S0140-6736(20)30964-8

Rehman, M., Khalid, F., Sheth, U., Al-Duaij, L., Chow, J., Azim, A., Last, N., Blissett, S., & Sibbald, M. (2024). Quarantining from professional identity: How did COVID-19 impact professional identity formation in undergraduate medical education? *Perspectives on Medical Education*, *13*(1), 130–140. https://doi.org/10.5334/pme.1308

Roberts, L. W. (2024). Women and academic medicine, 2020. *Academic Medicine: Journal of the Association of American Medical Colleges*, *95*(10), 1459–1464. https://doi.org/10.1097/ACM.0000000000003617

Sarkar, U., & Cassel, C. (2021). Humanism before heroism in medicine. *JAMA*, *326*(2), 127–128. https://doi.org/10.1001/jama.2021.9569

Sklar, D. P. (2020). COVID-19: Lessons from the disaster that can improve health professions education. *Academic Medicine*, *95*(11), 1631–3. https://doi.org/10.1097/ACM.0000000000003547

Skochelak, S. E., Lomis, K. D., Andrews, J. S., Hammoud, M. M., Mejicano, G. C., & Byerley, J. (2021). Realizing the vision of the Lancet Commission on education of health professionals for the 21st century: Transforming medical education through the accelerating change in medical education consortium. *Medical Teacher*, *43*(Suppl 2), S1–S6. https://doi.org/10.1080/0142159X.2021.1935833

Southworth, E., & Gleason, S. H. (2021). COVID 19: A cause for pause in undergraduate medical education and catalyst for innovation. *HEC Forum: An Interdisciplinary Journal on Hospitals' Ethical and Legal Issues*, *33*(1–2), 125–142. https://doi.org/10.1007/s10730-020-09433-5

Stetson, G. V., & Dhaliwal, G. (2021). Using a time out: Reimagining professional identity formation after the pandemic. *Medical Education*, *55*(1), 131–134. https://doi.org/10.1111/medu.14386

Triemstra, J. D., Haas, M. R. C., Bhavsar-Burke, I., Gottlieb-Smith, R., Wolff, M., Shelgikar, A. V., Samala, R. V., Ruff, A. L., Kuo, K., Tam, M., Gupta, A., Stojan, J., Gruppen, L., & Ellinas, H. (2021). Impact of the COVID-19 pandemic on the clinical learning environment: Addressing identified gaps and seizing opportunities. *Academic Medicine: Journal of the Association of American Medical Colleges*, *96*(9), 1276–1281. https://doi.org/10.1097/ACM.0000000000004013

Tsang, A. C. O., Shih, K. C., & Chen, J. Y. (2021). Clinical skills education at the bed-side, web-side and lab-side. *Medical Education*, *55*(1), 112–114. https://doi.org/10.1111/medu.14394

Wilensky, G. R. (2022, January 4). The COVID-19 pandemic and the US health care workforce. *JAMA Health Forum*, *3*(1), e220001. American Medical Association.

CHAPTER 9

Professional identity formation
Incorporating professionalism and care

....

Chest pain relieved by antacids: My last night as a resident

The astute intern standing next to me, noticing the beads of sweat forming on my forehead and my clenched fist rubbing my breastbone, walked to the medicine locker, grabbed a little blue bottle of antacid, and handed it to me. "If this works, I won't have to admit you on your last night on call as a resident!" he said cheerfully.

I slugged the chalky, mint flavored substance and almost immediately felt the chest pain—which I hadn't even fully noticed until then—resolve. "Thanks," I said, "You're gonna be a great resident in a few hours!" I glanced at my watch. *4 a.m. on June 30.* My last day as a house officer.

"1344 stat!" the crackling voice of the Bellevue Hospital operator cried from one of two cigarette-box-size beepers hanging off the waistband of my white pants. This dedicated "code beeper" was calling me to the emergency room where, luckily, I already was standing, ready to help my colleagues who were conducting a cardiac resuscitation on the patient in the "slot." This was not the cause of my heartburn. I loved this part. I was trained to do this, my movements were smooth and assured, the decision-making was practiced and honed. I felt competent and proud of my colleagues as we surrounded this patient, a man brought in by ambulance from Pennsylvania Station awake and alert, experiencing substernal chest pain and shortness of breath, who now needed us to save his life. And save his life we most likely would. This was quintessential doctoring, one patient at a time.

DOI: 10.1201/9781003507529-10

My heartburn was a result of the other beeper. The "medical consult" beeper was insisting, with the exact same urgency, that I call "bed board" (the office that managed the 400 adult beds in the hospital) and 17 West and 16 East and the Surgical ICU all at the same time. I added the callback numbers to the pink sheet on my clipboard. I made eye contact with the senior resident running the code to signal I was there if he needed me and picked up the wall phone.

This part of the job made my stomach acid churn. After a year of med consult calls, all of us senior residents had mastered—but did not have a positive attitude about—what we called the "hotel management" or "traffic cop" aspects of the job. We disliked assigning admitted patients to medical teams and working with the hospital administrator ("bed board") and nursing leadership to assign beds to those patients. It was a hard and thankless three-dimensional chess game. I didn't feel particularly good at or prepared for these logic puzzles. But I engaged because it was my job on the team that night.

There was also the "consultation" part of the job, which sounds like an opportunity to engage in erudite conversation with residents on other services about how to best care for patients, but that wasn't how things worked. The attending physicians did that part. Most often, we residents engaged in tense discussions demanding to transfer patients from their service to ours or vice versa. Too often, we debated whose "job" it was to adjust antibiotics or blood pressure medications. I would argue that *any* physician could handle this simple task with a little advice from us, but they would argue that their job was complete, and the patient now belonged on our team. We would argue where the patient with ominous abdominal pain should be monitored, our team contending that the physicians who could provide definitive surgical therapy would be best positioned to manage the patient, while they argued that until an intervention was needed, the patient should stay with us. On and on. Over and over.

Senior residents developed reputations of being a "wall," staving off patient transfers by playing expert, impenetrable defense; or of being a "sieve," easily persuaded to accept the transfer. I won't tell you which reputation I had, except to hint that I *did* accept transfers to our service only when it was obvious that a patient would be best cared for on our team. This was a judgment call, and I trusted both teams to do right by the patient.

It was also true that I didn't have the courage or tenacity to insist that other teams handle problems outside of their comfort zones. I have since gotten over that.

Physician professional identity formation, in those days, was in a very tribal stage of development. We worked in teams and, as teams, we defended our boundaries. As soon-to-be attending physicians, our main developmental challenge was balancing team loyalty and identity with a much more subtle discernment about "what is best for the patient." These situations were very complex; a single correct answer was unlikely. Beyond the formidable technical aspects of our disciplines, we attempted to discern what was really, holistically best for each patient right now and under these circumstances. Without realizing it at the time, we were developing the practical wisdom needed to thrive as a physician for a lifetime.

This critical learning process literally gave me chest pain.

Eventually, the new consult resident, in a fresh scrub shirt and white pants, came by to take over the beepers. She listened carefully to my recitation, jotting down the names, locations, and vital facts about the consults still to be seen and of those who needed follow-up. We reviewed the remaining "bed board" issues. I asked her to check on the freshly resuscitated patient; finding him a hospital bed was a priority. The resident had been at our class's graduation ceremony the week before, so she knew of my plans for a year abroad for medical education research and my ensuing fellowship. She wished me luck.

I found myself wistful and sentimental about her very first med consult shift and envious of her freshness and eagerness to do right and good. I hoped she would develop the wisdom needed to navigate the complexities in the best interests of our patients, without spending much time seriously considering being either a wall or a sieve. But we didn't have any time to discuss this, both beepers were already sounding.

I cleared out my locker and packed up the remaining books, toiletries, and other odds and ends. Gathering up fresh beeper batteries and a few single dose bottles of antacid I had pilfered from the nurse's station, I left them on the table in the on-call room. Someone would need them sooner rather than later.[1]

* * *

The clinician in this opening narrative experiences a major transition from resident to fellow. This last night on call in the resident role is a reflection, in a nutshell, of what the residency was all about. Now, a lifetime of a medical career is ahead of her, and her cart is packed with experiences, knowledge, skills, and an identity. Nevertheless, "Physician professional identity formation, in those days, was in a very tribal stage of development. We worked in teams and, as teams, we defended our boundaries. As soon-to-be attending physicians, our main developmental challenge was balancing team loyalty and identity with a much more subtle discernment about 'what is best for the patient.'"

---

1   Kalet, A. (2021, July 9). Chest pain relieved by antacids: My last night as a resident. *Transformational Times: Newsletter of the Robert D. and Patricia E. Kern Institute for the Transformation of Medical Education.*

PROFESSIONALIZATION AND PROFESSIONAL IDENTITY FORMATION

In the last two decades, a revised view on the becoming of a physician has gained prominence in the literature. There is agreement that becoming a physician is a self-altering process, described also as a "formation" (a term borrowed from clergy education) – a professional identity formation (PIF) journey. As previously mentioned, this relatively new outlook combines a critique of the different stage models suggested (categories 1–4) and makes room for reflection (category 5) with a fresher view of the professionalization process. Nevertheless, whether PIF truly integrates the issues of woundedness, racism, and discrimination, or the impact of the coronavirus pandemic and other external structural forces (categories 6–8), remains to be seen.

Cohen et al., who are psychoanalysts and psychiatrists and therefore in a position to bridge the psychoanalytically oriented first category with the present, final category, review the literature on the impact of medical school on personal development and consolidation of core identity.[2] In an article published in 2009, they claim that the limited literature relies on medical students' journaling exercises, discussion groups, post-graduation surveys, and repeated personality testing. They review forces acting on medical students, with potential transformational effects. These include high external expectations and internal fear of superficial knowledge and skills, entry into the culture of medicine with its insider jargon and hierarchy, high academic workload, and the emotional burdens of confronting cadavers and death as well as bearing witness to patient suffering. Potential developmental delay, emergence of substance abuse and hedonic acting out, cynicism, and loss of individual core values are possible consequences.

Weston has described that some students might exhaust all their developmental energies getting into and through training, to the extent that they skip some fundamental aspects of "growing up," e.g., Erikson's stage of identity vs. identity confusion, which then interferes with the next developmental stage of intimacy vs. isolation. Cohen et al. identify protections against these adverse potentialities, including identification of strong mentors and role models, developing postconventional morality and relativistic thinking, finding healthy coping strategies such

---

2   Cohen, M. J., Kay, A., Youakim, J. M., & Balaicuis, J. M. (2009). Identity transformation in medical students. *American Journal of Psychoanalysis*, 69(1), 43–52. https://doi.org/10.1057/ajp.2008.38

as peer support, and remaining intellectually creative and personally reflective. These protections underlie the social mechanisms—the professional community, mentors, and role models—that contribute to an individual's adaptability and resilience. **Hafferty** echoes Cohen et al., stating:

> Framing medical education as resocialization moves us from the seduction of imagining medical training as a simple augmentative or additive process in which a new set of occupationally specific knowledge, behaviors, and dispositions "simply" are layered onto previously existing ones. … [Doing so] forces us to view it as a more intentional, purposeful, and prescriptive social process whereby certain aspects of one's prior self are replaced by new ways of thinking, acting, and valuing.[3]
>
> (p. 61)

Webster-Wright characterizes the current view of PIF as a shift in focus from delivering and evaluating professional development programs to understanding and supporting authentic professional learning. Not only looking at what the professional knows and does, but also at who she is.[4] **Dall'Alba** reiterates Levinson's emphasis on ontology before epistemology (lived experience before its description and measurement),[5] writing that "at any given time there are not one but many different practices … [that vary] considerably across contexts. … Some variations may conflict with one another." Accordingly, she criticizes stage models as abstractions (epistemology) that ignore reality (ontology): while she applauds the contribution of the Dreyfus model, she states that it ignores the ways of being that are embodied and enacted in practice. She claims that when knowledge and skills are decontextualized from the practices to which they relate, integration is left to the learner, and that when only intellect is considered relevant, commitment, openness, wonder, and passion are lost. For Webster-Wright, Dall'Alba, and Levinson, knowledge is both

---

3   Hafferty, F. W. (2016). Socialization, professionalism, and professional identity formation. In R. L. Cruess, S. R. Cruess, & Y. Steinert (Eds.), *Teaching medical professionalism: Supporting the development of a professional identity* (pp. 54–67). Cambridge University Press.

4   Webster-Wright, A. (2009). Reframing professional development through understanding authentic professional learning. *Review of Educational Research*, 79(2), 702–739. https://doi.org/10.3102/0034654308330970

5   Dall'Alba, G. (2018). Reframing expertise and its development: A lifeworld perspective. In K. A. Ericsson, R. R. Hoffman, A. Kozbelt, & A. M. Williams (Eds.), *The Cambridge handbook of expertise and expert performance* (2nd ed., pp. 33–39). Cambridge University Press. https://doi.org/10.1017/9781316480748.003

situated and embodied. An alternative model she suggests includes a vertical axis representing **embodied understanding of practice** compared to **a horizontal axis representing skill progression**. Thus, **being is coupled with doing**.

Rees and Monrouxe[6] offer another view of identity and identification in medical education. Monrouxe asserts:

> Over the decades … this "internal" view [of the self] has been supplanted by the notion that identities are a product of intersubjective and external social processes. Identities are constructed and co-constructed as we participate in day-to-day social activities and through the use of language and artefacts and within power relations.[7]

Our primary embodied identities are those of gender, ethnicity, and social class. Consequently, when engaged in medical identity formation, **identity dissonance** may be behind, for example, the underperformance of women from disadvantaged sociocultural backgrounds and ethnic minorities.

Offering a personal view on becoming a medical professional, **Kirsty Foster** sees this becoming as "complex and multifaceted … an irreversible transformation. … The way that one feels about oneself and the way in which one interacts with the world are forever influenced by assuming the identity of 'doctor.'"[8] She describes an expansive process of knowledge and skill gaining accompanied by "bringing the learner in step … moving towards conformity" with the professional culture and societal expectations. Additionally, she refers to a paper by **Slotnick** and **Hilton**, who describe two key features in achieving phronesis: **experience and reflection on experience, and balance between attainment and attrition**.[9]

Goldie takes the bull of professional identity formation by the horns, adapting the Personality and Social Structure Perspective (PSSP) model

6   Rees, C. E., & Monrouxe, L. V. (2018). Who are you and who do you want to be? Key considerations in developing professional identities in medicine. *Medical Journal of Australia*, 209(5), 202–203. https://doi.org/10.5694/mja18.00118

7   Monrouxe, L. V. (2010). Identity, identification and medical education: Why should we care? *Medical Education*, 44(1), 40–49. https://doi.org/10.1111/j.1365-2923.2009.03440.x

8   Foster, K. (2011). Becoming a professional doctor. In L. Scanlon (Ed.), *"Becoming" a professional: An interdisciplinary analysis of professional learning* (pp. 171–193). Lifelong Learning Book Series, vol. 16. Springer. https://doi.org/10.1007/978-94-007-1378-9_9

9   Slotnick, H. B., & Hilton, S. R. (2006). Proto-professionalism and the dissecting laboratory. *Clinical Anatomy*, 19(5), 429–436. https://doi.org/10.1002/ca.20311

to inform a model of PIF, as well as sociopsychological levels of analysis applied to identity formation and identity maintenance processes.[10] He echoes the consensus that medical education is not only about acquiring competencies but also about developing a professional identity; that is, "ways of being and relating in professional contexts." Goldie suggests that "identity is multiple, dynamic, relational, situated, embedded in relations of power, yet negotiable."

Goldie asserts that personality and identity have the potential for change well into adulthood, refuting the myth that medical education and practice cannot transform a person or her identity, or that there is an age limit on developing as a healer. Echoing other scholars, Goldie states that meaning is created rather than transmitted and that culture is constantly recreated, a departure from deterministic views toward dynamic, co-creative ones. He classifies levels of student identity: the ego identity (Eriksonian), the personal one (meeting of the ego and social identities), and the social identity (shaped by relations and reflected to the student). He highlights the notion of **identity capital** (tangible and intangible) and expands upon multiple identities in operation as the core of the identification process.

Goldie then moves to the implications for educators, which include the need to interact with older professionals, especially role models and mentors, with attention to feedback provision; reflection and use of narratives; and, finally, **relational spaces** with patients and other health professionals. Throughout his paper, Goldie reiterates the complex nature of identity formation while inviting the formation of **identity complexity**.

As this book neared completion, **Sarraf-Yazdi** et al. published a graphic summary of PIF that aligns with the relational view of formation. Representing stages, stimuli, and responses, it includes an illustrated graph of a professional's perceived identity unfolding (diverging depending on whether she is supported or unsupported), and a lower row describing possible institutional involvement (Figure 9.1).[11]

---

10 Goldie, J. (2012). The formation of professional identity in medical students: Considerations for educators. *Medical Teacher*, 34(9), e641–e648. https://doi.org/10.3109/0142159X.2012.687476

11 Sarraf-Yazdi, S., Goh, S., & Krishna, L. (2024). Conceptualizing professional identity formation in medicine. *Academic Medicine: Journal of the Association of American Medical Colleges*, 99(3), 343. https://doi.org/10.1097/ACM.0000000000005559

Example	Medical Student	Resident/Trainee		Practicing Doctor		Life After Medicine
Event (STIMULUS)	Finds foundational sciences in first year lacking in clinical context.	Experiences discrimination due to ethnicity on the wards.	Loses a patient unexpectedly in final year of residency.	Works long hours during the pandemic with limited resources.	Receives a mid-career transition opportunity.	Retires from medical practice after decades.
Individual's Experience of Event (RESPONSE)	Loses motivation for medicine, is [not] able to seek guidance.	Feels angry and disillusioned, is [not] able to speak up.	Feels guilty and questions capabilities, does [not] have an opportunity to reflect with team under guidance.	Feels institutionally [un]supported, is [un]able to escape burnout.	Feels conflicted, is [not] able to seek out mentors to weigh options and make an informed decision.	Does [not] have diversified interests, is [not] able to find meaning beyond physician identity.

Aspirational

Perceived Identity

Existing

Trajectory is an aggregate of contextual modulations in response to events.

Same event can be experienced differently with/without support.

Supported ——
Unsupported - - -

Event

| Institution Promotes | Formal curriculum with clear and consistent learning and assessment goals pertaining to PIF. | Role models who uphold professional conduct, support psychological well-being, and foster reflection and inquiry. | Guided reflection opportunities as a social learning process to enable meaning-making of challenging or conflicting experiences. | Inclusive institutional mission and organizational culture open to dialogue, inquiry, equity, and improvement. | Mentoring capabilities to guide mentees on ways to navigate challenging professional experiences. | Self-care strategies to diversify interests early and mitigate a threat of declining self-efficacy, belonging, role continuity, or meaning. |

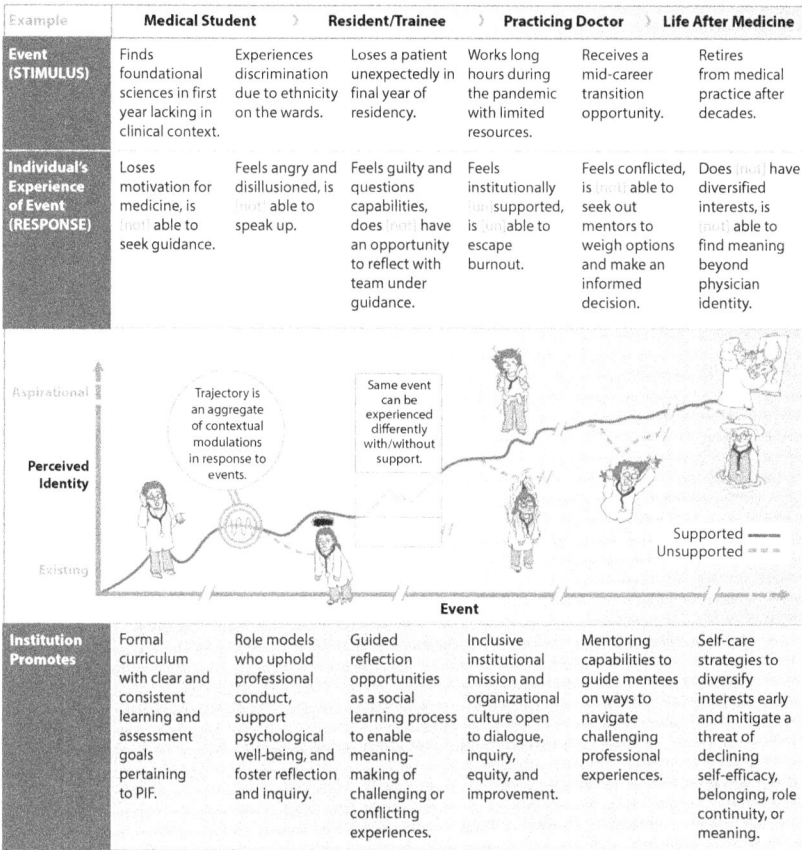

FIGURE 9.1 Conceptualizing Professional Identity Formation in Medicine (From Sarraf-Yazdi 2024. Reproduced with permission from the Copyright Clearance Center.)

Jarvis-Selinger et al. agree that competency discourse should be complemented with an identity discourse.[12] They reiterate two levels on which a medical learner's identity is shaped: the personal and the social. Further, they posit the construct of "role" in between competence and identity, emphasizing that **a role is a space in which competence and identity interact.** Thus, being in the role of a resident, for

---

12 Jarvis-Selinger, S., Pratt, D. D., & Regehr, G. (2012). Competency is not enough: Integrating identity formation into the medical education discourse. Academic Medicine: Journal of the Association of American Medical Colleges, 87(9), 1185–1190. https://doi.org/10.1097/ACM.0b013e3182604968

instance, defines expected competences and an identity which is not only a developmental stage on the way to becoming an independent practitioner, but is that of "resident." Moving to the next stage will not only consist of acquiring the identity of a board-certified physician but also of giving up the identity of a resident—a shift accompanied by a new learning environment and a different tension between service and learning associated with the new identity, as illustrated in this chapter's opening story.

Further, Jarvis-Selinger et al. quote Kegan as a salient example of developmental theorists who address individual identity formation, with **a crisis as the "crucible" of each required transition, in which increased vulnerability and heightened potential exist.** Elaborating on the influences of social context on identity formation, they write: "It is the connection to these specific communities of practice that gives meaning to the formation and expression of identities." Consequently, competence needs to be aligned with role and the process of identity formation, and these need to be coordinated. Finally, Jarvis-Selinger et al. call for replacing competency frameworks (e.g., CanMEDS and ACGME), which have an implicit linear assumption, with the discontinuous one offered by developmental theorists.

Chandran et al. echo the former scholars by suggesting pedagogies that foster "ways of being" rather than only competencies.[13] They write that Dall'Alba, Monrouxe, Goldie, and Jarvis-Selinger et al. are advancing the discourse on physician formation by offering integrative, nuanced, complex, and inclusive views that include individual and social components and forces. Moreover, they also resonate with the work of **Cooke** et al.[14] on reform of medical school and residency, who placed a decisive emphasis on formation and identity. Cooke et al. identify within present professional formation a lack of clarity and focus on professional values, inadequate expectations for progressively higher levels of professional commitment, failure to assess, and erosion in values. In turn, they suggest promoting formal ethics instruction, storytelling, and the use of symbols (honor codes, pledges, white coat ceremonies), as well as addressing the hidden curriculum. They highlight offering feedback and opportunities for reflection and assessment

---

13 Chandran, L., Iuli, R. J., Strano-Paul, L., & Post, S. G. (2019). Developing "a way of being": Deliberate approaches to professional identity formation in medical education. *Academic Psychiatry: The Journal of the American Association of Directors of Psychiatric Residency Training and the Association for Academic Psychiatry, 43*(5), 521–527. https://doi.org/10.1007/s40596-019-01048-4

14 Cooke, M., Irby, D. M., & O'Brien, B. C. (2010). Educating physicians: *A call for reform of medical school and residency.* Jossey-Bass.

of professionalism in the context of longitudinal mentoring and advising, asserting that "without a forum to share and reflect on their moral choices, students feel isolated and unable to resolve their identity and ethical conflict."

Further, Cooke et al. reiterate that **learning involves the construction of identities**. They describe the way in which opportunities to push boundaries of knowledge and understanding are core to development, and how progress in clinical reasoning frees up mental space to accommodate growing complexity (see the "crucible of learning" in Chapter 10). **Kelly** identifies developing the capacity for **resilience and forgiveness** as additional features of growth.[15]

For Bleakley et al.,[16] to become a doctor or another health professional is to take on an identity or a compound of identities associated with multiple roles. They emphasize, like others cited earlier, that the vicissitudes of a medical identity are intimately associated with power and suggest a formula, **identity × power × location (place, context) × uncertainty (patients)**, as the calculus of the transition from **critical reasoning to practical reasoning (phronesis)**. They claim the following:

> Forms of *power* are at play that lead to the legitimization (and then adoption) of certain ways of doing things, while making other possible ways illegitimate, which are then excluded. ... "Adult learning theory" ... characterized by emphasis upon the "autonomous learner," "self-directed learning" and "self-assessment"—is not a *natural* or *best* way to do learning, but is a product of ideology, itself a condition of power. ... Learning is then fundamentally political. But learning and education are also intimately tied with two other issues besides power: *identity* and *location* (or place).

Thus, Bleakley et al. invite a discourse on how power and location also shape developmental practices and trajectories, and challenge traditional methods as inadequate for the present and future directions of healthcare, medical education, and PIF. As our analysis has already shown, external forces such as political systems, socioeconomics, and natural and man-made disasters create contexts that shape learning and identity

---

15 Kelly, J. D., 4th. (2018). Forgiveness: A key resiliency builder. *Clinical Orthopaedics and Related Research*, 476(2), 203–204. https://doi.org/10.1007/s11999 .0000000000000024

16 Bleakley, A., Bligh, J., & Browne, J. (2011). *Medical education for the future: Identity, power and location.* Springer.

formation, at times surpassing the noble intentions and pedagogies of medical educators.

Echoing Bleakley et al. and **Mokhachane** et al.,[17] **Helmich** et al.[18] advocate for a context-specific approach to professional identity formation. In doing so, they aim to broaden the developing PIF discourse to also include non-Western approaches and notions.[19]

KEGAN'S BRIDGE METAPHOR

Lewin et al.[20] investigate Kegan's adult development model (see Chapter 1), albeit from the PIF perspective. They write:

> Building on Kegan's bridge metaphor, we have come to think of being in this transformational space as traversing a bridge as one builds it, the near end anchored in the traveler's current form of mind with its familiar lens and the far end in a foreign-feeling but objectively definable place. This process occurs in fits and starts, and persons frequently spend as much time on the bridge as on either side. Knowing this sheds a different light on our responsibility as educators to respond with empathy to learners who are tempted to retreat to more comfortable ways of knowing and to support their growth by acknowledging their journey and assuring them we believe they can get to the other side.

This metaphor also suggests the possibility of getting stuck in between, having forgone a comfort zone, identity, role, and competence without

17 Mokhachane, M., George, A., Wyatt, T., Kuper, A., & Green-Thompson, L. (2023). Rethinking professional identity formation amidst protests and social upheaval: A journey in Africa. *Advances in Health Sciences Education: Theory and Practice, 28*(2), 427–452. https://doi.org/10.1007/s10459-022-10164-0

18 Helmich, E., Yeh, H. M., Yeh, C. C., de Vries, J., Fu-Chang Tsai, D., & Dornan, T. (2017). Emotional learning and identity development in medicine: A cross-cultural qualitative study comparing Taiwanese and Dutch medical undergraduates. *Academic Medicine: Journal of the Association of American Medical Colleges, 92*(6), 853–859. https://doi.org/10.1097/ACM.0000000000001658

19 Cruess, R. L., Cruess, S. R., Boudreau, J. D., Snell, L., & Steinert, Y. (2015). A schematic representation of the professional identity formation and socialization of medical students and residents: A guide for medical educators. *Academic Medicine: Journal of the Association of American Medical Colleges, 90*(6), 718–725. https://doi.org/10.1097/ACM.0000000000000700

20 Lewin, L. O., McManamon, A., Stein, M. T. O., & Chen, D. T. (2019). Minding the form that transforms: Using Kegan's model of adult development to understand personal and professional identity formation in medicine. *Academic Medicine: Journal of the Association of American Medical Colleges, 94*(9), 1299–1304. https://doi.org/10.1097/ACM.0000000000002741

having fully reached new versions of these at the other end of the "bridge." This is sometimes termed in the literature as a "split" stance, as in the split psychosocial model used to describe a practitioner who has already given up her attachment to the biomedical model but has not yet reached a full commitment to and practice of the biopsychosocial model.[21,22,23] Such a state also echoes the constructs of the zone of proximal development (ZPD) and liminality (which we have called the "crucible of learning"; see Chapter 10).

Furthermore, Lewin et al. add:

> We see this model informing many aspects of medical education, from admissions and grading policies to curriculum development, remediation, and academic advising. We believe that taking Kegan's ideas into account can also provide new perspectives on, and deepen the conversations around, milestones, competencies, and entrustable professional activities. Further, this model can guide leadership development, as oversight of our complex adaptive health systems in an environment of volatility, uncertainty, complexity, and ambiguity likely requires individuals who have begun to develop *self-transforming* minds.

PROFESSIONALISM, COMPETENCY-BASED MEDICAL EDUCATION, AND PROFESSIONAL IDENTITY FORMATION

Cruess et al. have linked professionalism with PIF in the second edition of their seminal book on teaching professionalism. Throughout the book, a host of distinguished scholars effectively argue that PIF is the aim of medical education, supporting this stance with evidence, theory, and case studies, and proposing possible evaluation modalities. To achieve this aim, however, present-day scholars urge an empirical inquiry into these scholarly claims, which still lack a solid research base. Others proclaim that transformative learning, master adaptive learning, and practical wisdom are the ultimate goals of physician formation.

21 Biderman, A., Yeheskel, A., & Herman, J. (2005). The biopsychosocial model—have we made any progress since 1977? *Families, Systems, & Health, 23*(4), 379–386. https://doi.org/10.1037/1091-7527.23.4.379

22 Epstein, R. M., & Borrell-Carrio, F. (2005). The biopsychosocial model: Exploring six impossible things. *Families, Systems, & Health, 23*(4), 426–431. https://doi.org/10.1037/1091-7527.23.4.426

23 Weston, W. W. (2005). Patient-centered medicine: A guide to the biopsychosocial model. *Families, Systems, & Health, 23*(4), 387–392. https://doi.org/10.1037/1091-7527.23.4.387

Cruess et al. represent PIF and its associated socialization in graphic form and detail the conditions needed to support it[24] (Figures 9.2–9.4).In Figure 9.2, they mention learning the language and learning to live with uncertainty, as well as learning the hierarchy and power relationships that feed into learning to "play the role." This is how socialization is put in motion. Both negative influences (such as cynicism or stress) and positive ones (such as increased competence and satisfaction) interact while the process adds the professional identity to the personal identity.

In Figure 9.3, the factors involved in socialization are represented: personal context, learning environment, and the healthcare system, alongside formal teaching, symbols, and rituals. These elements play a role that feeds into experiences, role models, and mentoring, which in turn are processed through conscious reflection and unconscious acquisition.

Figure 9.4 focuses on PIF. "Who you are" undergoes negotiation during socialization, with acceptance, compromise, or rejection of a

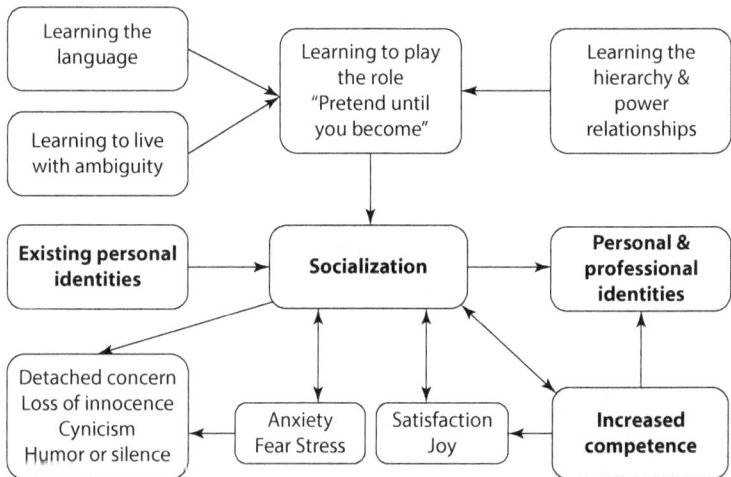

FIGURE 9.2 A Schematic Representation of the Roles Medical Students and Residents Play during the Process of Socialization and Their Potential Response to This Process (From Cruess et al. 2015. Reproduced with permission from the Copyright Clearance Center.)

24 Cruess, R. L., Cruess, S. R., Boudreau, J. D., Snell, L., & Steinert, Y. (2014). Reframing medical education to support professional identity formation. *Academic Medicine: Journal of the Association of American Medical Colleges*, 89(11), 1446–1451. https://doi.org/10.1097/ACM.0000000000000427

myriad of identity facets to shape "Who you become." This individual process is embedded in the movement from the periphery of the community of practice to full participation in it.

Multiple additional authors have been writing about the multitude of aspects that constitute PIF, including its measurement.[25,26,27,28,29,30,31,32,33,34] These include **Sternszus** et al., who have recently described three contradictions between the paradigms of competency-based medical education (CBME) and PIF, suggesting ways to reconcile them:

25 Cruess, S. R., Cruess, R. L., & Steinert, Y. (2019). Supporting the development of a professional identity: General principles. *Medical Teacher, 41*(6), 641–649. https://doi.org/10.1080/0142159X.2018.1536260

26 Lawrence, E. C., Carvour, M. L., Camarata, C., Andarsio, E., & Rabow, M. W. (2020). Requiring the healer's art curriculum to promote professional identity formation among medical students. *Journal of Medical Humanities, 41*(4), 531–541. https://doi.org/10.1007/s10912-020-09649-z

27 Cruess, R. L., Cruess, S. R., & Steinert, Y. (2016). Amending Miller's pyramid to include professional identity formation. *Academic Medicine: Journal of the Association of American Medical Colleges, 91*(2), 180–185. https://doi.org/10.1097/ACM.0000000000000913

28 Johnston, S. (2006). See one, do one, teach one: Developing professionalism across the generations. *Clinical Orthopaedics and Related Research, 449*, 186–192. https://doi.org/10.1097/01.blo.0000224033.23850.1c

29 Adema, M., Dolmans, D. H. J. M., Raat, J. A. N., Scheele, F., Jaarsma, A. D. C., & Helmich, E. (2019). Social interactions of clerks: The role of engagement, imagination, and alignment as sources for professional identity formation. *Academic Medicine: Journal of the Association of American Medical Colleges, 94*(10), 1567–1573. https://doi.org/10.1097/ACM.0000000000002781

30 Tagawa, M. (2019). Development of a scale to evaluate medical professional identity formation. *BMC Medical Education, 19*(1), 63. https://doi.org/10.1186/s12909-019-1499-9

31 Nothnagle, M., Reis, S., Goldman, R. E., & Anandarajah, G. (2014). Fostering professional formation in residency: Development and evaluation of the "forum" seminar series. *Teaching and Learning in Medicine, 26*(3), 230–238. https://doi.org/10.1080/10401334.2014.910124

32 Yiu, S., Yeung, M., Cheung, W. J., & Frank, J. R. (2023). Stress and conflict from tacit culture forges professional identity in newly graduated independent physicians. *Advances in Health Sciences Education: Theory and Practice, 28*(3), 847–870. https://doi.org/10.1007/s10459-022-10173-z

33 Veen, M., & de la Croix, A. (2023). How to grow a professional identity: Philosophical gardening in the field of medical education. *Perspectives on Medical Education, 12*(1), 12–19. https://doi.org/10.5334/pme.367

34 Mount, G. R., Kahlke, R., Melton, J., & Varpio, L. (2022). A critical review of professional identity formation interventions in medical education. *Academic Medicine: Journal of the Association of American Medical Colleges, 97*(11S), S96–S106. https://doi.org/10.1097/ACM.0000000000004904

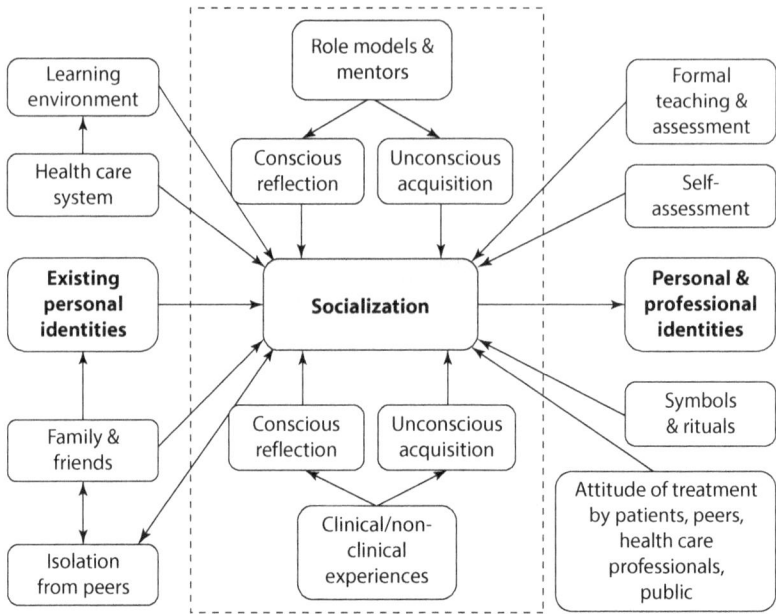

FIGURE 9.3 A Schematic Representation of the Multiple Factors Involved in the Process of Socialization in Medicine (From Cruess et al. 2015. Reproduced with permission from the Copyright Clearance Center.)

[There are] three contradictions that must and can be resolved, namely: (1) CBME attends to behavioral outcomes whereas PIF attends to developmental processes; (2) CBME emphasizes standardization whereas PIF emphasizes individualization; (3) CBME organizes assessment around observed competence whereas the assessment of PIF is inherently more holistic. Subsequently, the authors identify curricular opportunities to address these contradictions, such as incorporating process-based outcomes into curricula, recognizing the individualized and contextualized nature of competence, and incorporating guided self-assessment into coaching and mentorship programs. In addition, the authors highlight future research directions related to each contradiction with the goal of reconciling "doing" and "being" in medical education.[35]

35 Sternszus, R., Slattery, N. K., Cruess, R. L., Cate, O. T., Hamstra, S. J., & Steinert, Y. (2023). Contradictions and opportunities: Reconciling professional identity formation and competency-based medical education. *Perspectives on Medical Education*, 12(1), 507–516. https://doi.org/10.5334/pme.1027

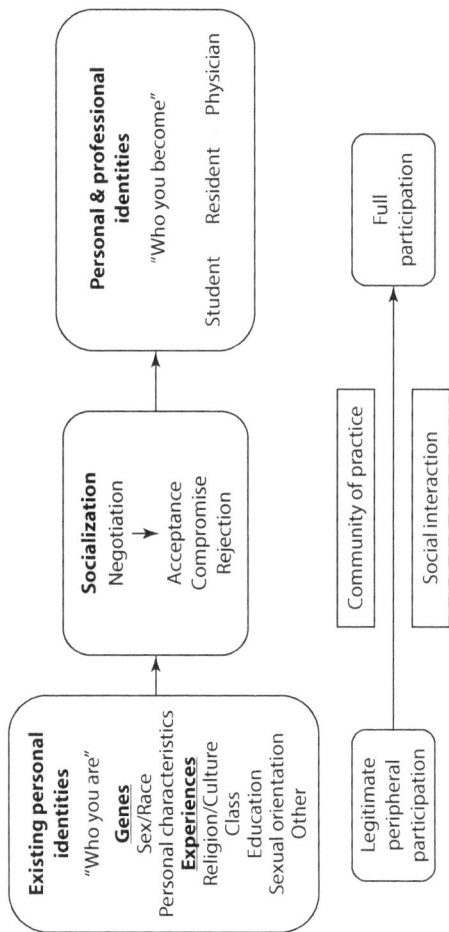

FIGURE 9.4 A Schematic Representation of Professional Identity Formation (From Cruess et al. 2015. Reproduced with permission from the Copyright Clearance Center.)

CARE AND PROFESSIONAL IDENTITY FORMATION

Kleinman's *The Soul of Care*[36] is about **caring about others, being careful, and caring for others**. As his ailing wife's primary caregiver, he was summoned to embody his morality, values, and love. He writes:

> I think of care as first and foremost a developmental process that, whatever its biological basis, is learned and practised as part of personal development, social cultivation, and maturation of our sensibilities and capabilities. ... Our cares ... clarify what is, experientially, most at stake for each of us: responding to pain and suffering, enduring the unendurable, living lives of purpose and meaning, building and maintaining relations with others who are close to us, doing work that sustains us and matters, taking care of the environment and community around us. ... When one of us is sick or disabled we expect, or at least hope, that care will be forthcoming. It is a learned assumption, though not always fulfilled, about how families and communities will and should behave.
>
> Care is an embodied experience for both the caregiver and receiver. Caring acts are centred on physical acts of touching, embracing, steadying, lifting, toileting, and so on. But they also include the way we look at someone and receive their return gaze; the way we connect (or fail to do so); the quality of our voice, our very presence. All contribute a particular caring tone, or its absence. Theories ... deepen our understanding of care as a form of "doing" or a mode of "acting" on different levels and in different registers: more verb than noun.[37]

Kleinman's profound message is shockingly simple. Medicine is one expression of the vast world of care. However, it is in a deep crisis of care, along with our entire society.[38] He calls, as several others do, for the incorporation of care experiences into the fabric of medical training and the revolutionization of care in healthcare. Thus, Kleinman advocates developing caregiving as part of and in addition to the professional and personal development of physicians.

---

36 Kleinman, A. (2019). *The soul of care: The moral education of a husband and doctor.* Viking.

37 Kleinman, A. (2015). Care: In search of a health agenda. *Lancet, 386*(9990), 240–241. https://doi.org/10.1016/S0140-6736(15)61271-5

38 Kleinman, A. (2020). Varieties of experiences of care. *Perspectives in Biology and Medicine, 63*(3), 458–465. https://doi.org/10.1353/pbm.2020.0033

Adding to the discourse on competence versus identity, **MacLeod** highlights the tension between discourses on competence and care in medical education.[39] She describes:

> Professional identities are developed in relation to discourses of competence, ... students displayed what they considered to be desirable professional identities of confidence, capability and suitability. Also explored are the professional identities demonstrated in relation to discourses of caring, including those of benevolence and humbleness.

Caregiving is not confined to doctors, nor to health professionals. While largely ignored by classical scholars, comprehensive theories of care began to emerge in the early 1980s, proposed by philosophers such as **Nel Noddings**[40] and **Joan Tronto**,[41] and psychologists such as Carol Gilligan, who argue that caring is the foundation of morality. Caregiving is what countless parents (primarily mothers) and caregivers (mostly women) practice daily. The additional burden of care that female physicians shoulder once they are parenting or caretaking must be acknowledged. However, the psychology and philosophy of care may need to be revisited and extended to support the formation of a physician's identity.

LIMINALITY AND FURTHER INTEGRATION

Elaborating on liminality and identity work, Gordon et al.[42,43] (also discussed in Chapter 1) assert the complexity of transition and identity work. They suggest that the "occupying of liminal spaces, as our data illustrate, allowed our participants time to make sense of his or her developing identities," and that "our study findings ... [are] illustrating doctors' narrations of *perpetual* liminality and occupying liminality,

39 MacLeod, A. (2011). Caring, competence and professional identities in medical education. *Advances in Health Sciences Education: Theory and Practice, 16*(3), 375–394. https://doi.org/10.1007/s10459-010-9269-9

40 Noddings, N. (1984). *Caring: A feminine approach to ethics and moral education.* University of California Press.

41 Tronto, J. C. (1993). *Moral boundaries: A political argument for an ethic of care.* Routledge. https://doi.org/10.4324/9781003070672

42 Gordon, L., Rees, C. E., & Jindal-Snape, D. (2020). Doctors' identity transitions: Choosing to occupy a state of 'betwixt and between'. *Medical Education, 54*(11), 1006–1018. https://doi.org/10.1111/medu.14219

43 Gordon, L., Teunissen, P. W., Jindal-Snape, D., Bates, J., Rees, C. E., Westerman, M., Sinha, R., & van Dijk, A. (2020). An international study of trainee-trained transitions: Introducing the transition-to-trained-doctor (T3D) model. *Medical Teacher, 42*(6), 679–688. https://doi.org/10.1080/0142159X.2020.1733508

and offering a more complex and multidimensional picture of transitions than has been presented previously."

Most of the categories we have identified in this book find a home and seem integrated into the current literature on professional identity formation. Also, many of the constructs in this chapter have already been introduced in former categories. Stages have become more complex and nuanced, evolving from simple or complicated portrayals to complex adaptive system modeling. An up-to-date understanding of individual adult learning has been incorporated into the communities of practice construct. Mentoring, coaching, and role modeling reside side by side with a view of expertise development through deliberate practice culminating in phronesis. Moral development, also complex and nuanced, moves toward the daily moral experience and its gap from the moral ideal, extending an invitation to include caregiving as an additional layer of humanity.[44] Narrative is extensively used to support reflection, self-awareness, professionalism, and sense-making of the journey.[45,46,47,48,49] Recognition of failures as well as triumphs throughout the physician life cycle lends a realistic bend to the inquiry, acknowledging error, regret, and developmental arrests as ubiquitous and frequently defining elements of personal and professional development. Embodiment, coping with strong emotions,[50] benevolence, humbleness, enduring the unen-

---

44 Shubkin, C. D., Garrett, J. R., & Lantos, J. D. (2018). When residents let conscience be their guide: Professional development and educational opportunity. *Academic Pediatrics, 18*(3), 239–242. https://doi.org/10.1016/j.acap.2017.12.003

45 Rees, C. E., Kent, F., & Crampton, P. E. S. (2019). Student and clinician identities: How are identities constructed in interprofessional narratives? *Medical Education, 53*(8), 808–823. https://doi.org/10.1111/medu.13886

46 Hatem, D. S., & Halpin, T. (2019). Becoming doctors: Examining student narratives to understand the process of professional identity formation within a learning community. *Journal of Medical Education and Curricular Development, 6.* https://doi.org/10.1177/2382120519834546

47 Morgan, A., Moore, J., & Duff, A. (2019). Guide the ways Tutored reflection facilitates professional identity formation. *Medical Teacher, 41*(2), 235–236. https://doi.org/10.1080/0142159X.2018.1515478

48 Wald, H. S., White, J., Reis, S. P., Esquibel, A. Y., & Anthony, D. (2019). Grappling with complexity: Medical students' reflective writings about challenging patient encounters as a window into professional identity formation. *Medical Teacher, 41*(2), 152–160. https://doi.org/10.1080/0142159X.2018.1475727

49 Branch, W. T., Jr, & Frankel, R. (2016). Not all stories of professional identity formation are equal: An analysis of formation narratives of highly humanistic physicians. *Patient Education and Counseling, 99*(8), 1394–1399. https://doi.org/10.1016/j.pec.2016.03.018

50 Lönn, A., Weurlander, M., Seeberger, A., Hult, H., Thornberg, R., & Wernerson, A. (2023). The impact of emotionally challenging situations on medical students' professional identity formation. *Advances in Health Sciences Education: Theory and Practice, 28*(5), 1557–1578. https://doi.org/10.1007/s10459-023-10229-8

durable, living lives of purpose and meaning, building and maintaining relationships, doing what matters and is sustaining, and taking care of one's community complement the many complex and nuanced features suggested for proper PIF.

However, as already mentioned, critics raise the concern of bias in PIF literature since gender and race, as well as non-Western cultures, are relatively ignored. Similarly, the impact of external structural forces on the becoming and being of physicians has not been adequately acknowledged. This is most dramatically evident in the experiences of physicians under totalitarian regimes, in war zones, and/or within humanitarian disasters where survival comes first and professionalism, PIF, and morality may be deprioritized—or, as is sometimes the case, these situations can also be the source of remarkable heroism. This aspect of medical PIF is not yet fully described, recognized, or understood.

CRITICS OF PROFESSIONALISM AND PROFESSIONAL IDENTITY FORMATION CONSTRUCTS

Critics of the current view on PIF, such as **Wyatt** et al., are concerned that "the fact that race and ethnicity have been largely absent, invisible or considered irrelevant within PIF research is problematic."[51] The latter assert:

> Any attempt to explore professional identity is incomplete without also considering that a trainee's evolving sense of self is inexorably bound up with forces of knowledge, power, and ethics that shape them into becoming certain kinds of physician subjects rather than others. ... A genealogical approach determines how we reached the now in which we find ourselves and how we might transform it, such that we may shift the possibilities afforded to health professionals to establish professional identities aligned with their personal identities in ways that maximize inclusivity and minimize marginalization.

---

51 Wyatt, T. R., Balmer, D., Rockich-Winston, N., Chow, C. J., Richards, J., & Zaidi, Z. (2021). 'Whispers and shadows': A critical review of the professional identity literature with respect to minority physicians. *Medical Education*, 55, 148–158. https://doi.org/10.1111/medu.14295

Finally, race, gender, and marginalization (power relations) are brought into this discourse.[52,53,54] As we move our gaze in this direction, it becomes evident that woundedness and developmental challenges in the doctor's life cycle (DLC) are compounded for women and minorities. These issues have been further amplified by the pandemic.[55,56]

Ideally, models that allow us to see the ways in which minoritized identities, and in fact all personal identities, enhance and enrich PIF will be developed. The discourse that acknowledges these challenges is relatively new. How we might integrate its insights into our understanding of PIF remains a work in progress.

Summary

The opening story is about another DLC transition: the last day of residency. The narrator sheds a role and identity before she can assume the next role and identity she aspires to. This transition is abrupt in the moment and takes longer to process and assume the new role at the other end of the bridge.

The PIF construct integrates most of the earlier categories. Through the sophisticated elaboration of many scholars, a complex, nuanced, and widely accepted model has emerged. However, if our narrator was going through her transition, this liminality, in 2024, she would have probably added in her gendered challenges, her context, including politics, as well as how the pandemic impacted this transition. In other words, if we are to support PIF as the organizing construct for the DLC, we need to further explore how the doctor integrates new realities and both predictable and unpredictable challenges of adult life into the ongoing process of becoming a physician. This will be described in Chapter 10.

52 Trevino, R., & Poitevien, P. (2021). Professional identity formation for underrepresented in medicine learners. *Current Problems in Pediatric and Adolescent Health Care*, 51(10), 101091. https://doi.org/10.1016/j.cppeds.2021.101091

53 Fyfe, M., Horsburgh, J., Blitz, J., Chiavaroli, N., Kumar, S., & Cleland, J. (2022). The do's, don'ts and don't knows of redressing differential attainment related to race/ethnicity in medical schools. *Perspectives on Medical Education*, 11(1), 1–14. https://doi.org/10.1007/s40037-021-00696-3

54 Yu, C., Liu, Q., Wang, W., Xie, A., & Liu, J. (2022). Professional identity of 0.24 million medical students in China before and during the COVID-19 pandemic: Three waves of national cross-sectional studies. *Frontiers in Public Health*, 10, 868914. https://doi.org/10.3389/fpubh.2022.868914

55 Matsui, T., Sato, M., Kato, Y., & Nishigori, H. (2019). Professional identity formation of female doctors in Japan—Gap between the married and unmarried. *BMC Medical Education*, 19(1), 55. https://doi.org/10.1186/s12909-019-1479-0

56 Ranasinghe, P. D., & Zhou, A. (2023). Women physicians and the COVID-19 pandemic: Gender-based impacts and potential interventions. *Annals of Medicine*, 55(1), 319–324. https://doi.org/10.1080/07853890.2022.2164046

REFERENCES

Adema, M., Dolmans, D. H. J. M., Raat, J. A. N., Scheele, F., Jaarsma, A. D. C., & Helmich, E. (2019). Social interactions of clerks: The role of engagement, imagination, and alignment as sources for professional identity formation. *Academic Medicine: Journal of the Association of American Medical Colleges*, 94(10), 1567–1573. https://doi.org/10.1097/ACM.0000000000002781

Biderman, A., Yeheskel, A., & Herman, J. (2005). The biopsychosocial model—have we made any progress since 1977? *Families, Systems, & Health*, 23(4), 379–386. https://doi.org/10.1037/1091-7527.23.4.379

Bleakley, A., Bligh, J., & Browne, J. (2011). *Medical education for the future: Identity, power and location*. Springer

Branch, W. T., Jr, & Frankel, R. (2016). Not all stories of professional identity formation are equal: An analysis of formation narratives of highly humanistic physicians. *Patient Education and Counseling*, 99(8), 1394–1399. https://doi.org/10.1016/j.pec.2016.03.018

Chandran, L., Iuli, R. J., Strano-Paul, L., & Post, S. G. (2019). Developing "a way of being": Deliberate approaches to professional identity formation in medical education. *Academic Psychiatry: The Journal of the American Association of Directors of Psychiatric Residency Training and the Association for Academic Psychiatry*, 43(5), 521–527. https://doi.org/10.1007/s40596-019-01048-4

Cohen, M. J., Kay, A., Youakim, J. M., & Balaicuis, J. M. (2009). Identity transformation in medical students. *American Journal of Psychoanalysis*, 69(1), 43–52. https://doi.org/10.1057/ajp.2008.38.

Cooke, M., Irby, D. M., & O'Brien, B. (2010). *Educating physicians: A call for reform of medical school and residency*. Jossey-Bass.

Cruess, R. L., Cruess, S. R., Boudreau, J. D., Snell, L., & Steinert, Y. (2014). Reframing medical education to support professional identity formation. *Academic Medicine: Journal of the Association of American Medical Colleges*, 89(11), 1446–1451. https://doi.org/10.1097/ACM.0000000000000427

Cruess, R. L., Cruess, S. R., Boudreau, J. D., Snell, L., & Steinert, Y. (2015). A schematic representation of the professional identity formation and socialization of medical students and residents: A guide for medical educators. *Academic Medicine: Journal of the Association of American Medical Colleges*, 90(6), 718–725. https://doi.org/10.1097/ACM.0000000000000700

Cruess, R. L., Cruess, S. R., & Steinert, Y. (2016). Amending Miller's pyramid to include professional identity formation. *Academic Medicine: Journal of the Association of American Medical Colleges*, 91(2), 180–185. https://doi.org/10.1097/ACM.0000000000000913

Cruess, S. R., Cruess, R. L., & Steinert, Y. (2019). Supporting the development of a professional identity: General principles. *Medical Teacher*, 41(6), 641–649. https://doi.org/10.1080/0142159X.2018.1536260

Dall'Alba, G. (2018). Reframing expertise and its development: A lifeworld perspective. In K. A. Ericsson, R. R. Hoffman, A. Kozbelt, & A. M. Williams (Eds.), *The Cambridge handbook of expertise and expert performance* (2nd ed., pp. 33–39). Cambridge University Press. https://doi.org/10.1017/9781316480748.003

Epstein, R. M., & Borrell-Carrio, F. (2005). The biopsychosocial model: Exploring six impossible things. *Families, Systems, & Health*, 23(4), 426–431. https://doi.org/10.1037/1091-7527.23.4.426

Foster, K. (2011). Becoming a professional doctor. In L. Scanlon (Ed.), *"Becoming" a professional: An interdisciplinary analysis of professional learning* (Vol. 16, pp. 171–193). Lifelong Learning Book Series. Springer. https://doi.org/10.1007/978-94-007-1378-9_9

Fyfe, M., Horsburgh, J., Blitz, J., Chiavaroli, N., Kumar, S., & Cleland, J. (2022). The do's, don'ts and don't knows of redressing differential attainment related to race/ethnicity in medical schools. *Perspectives on Medical Education*, *11*(1), 1–14. https://doi.org/10.1007/s40037-021-00696-3

Goldie, J. (2012). The formation of professional identity in medical students: Considerations for educators. *Medical Teacher*, *34*(9), e641–e648. https://doi.org/10.3109/0142159X.2012.687476

Gordon, L., Rees, C. E., & Jindal-Snape, D. (2020). Doctors' identity transitions: Choosing to occupy a state of 'betwixt and between'. *Medical Education*, *54*(11), 1006–1018. https://doi.org/10.1111/medu.14219

Gordon, L., Teunissen, P. W., Jindal-Snape, D., Bates, J., Rees, C. E., Westerman, M., Sinha, R., & van Dijk, A. (2020). An international study of trainee-trained transitions: Introducing the transition-to-trained-doctor (T3D) model. *Medical Teacher*, *42*(6), 679–688. https://doi.org/10.1080/0142159X.2020.1733508

Hafferty, F. W. (2016). Socialization, professionalism, and professional identity formation. In R. L. Cruess, S. R. Cruess, & Y. Steinert (Eds.), *Teaching medical professionalism: Supporting the development of a professional identity* (pp. 54–67). Cambridge University Press.

Hatem, D. S., & Halpin, T. (2019). Becoming doctors: Examining student narratives to understand the process of professional identity formation within a learning community. *Journal of Medical Education and Curricular Development*, *6*. https://doi.org/10.1177/2382120519834546

Helmich, E., Yeh, H. M., Yeh, C. C., de Vries, J., Fu-Chang Tsai, D., & Dornan, T. (2017). Emotional learning and identity development in medicine: A cross-cultural qualitative study comparing Taiwanese and Dutch medical undergraduates. *Academic Medicine: Journal of the Association of American Medical Colleges*, *92*(6), 853–859. https://doi.org/10.1097/ACM.0000000000001658

Jarvis-Selinger, S., Pratt, D. D., & Regehr, G. (2012). Competency is not enough: Integrating identity formation into the medical education discourse. *Academic Medicine: Journal of the Association of American Medical Colleges*, *87*(9), 1185–1190. https://doi.org/10.1097/ACM.0b013e3182604968

Johnston, S. (2006). See one, do one, teach one: Developing professionalism across the generations. *Clinical Orthopaedics and Related Research*, *449*, 186–192. https://doi.org/10.1097/01.blo.0000224033.23850.1c

Kalet, A. (2021, July 9). Chest pain relieved by antacids: My last night as a resident. *Transformational Times: Newsletter of the Robert D. and Patricia E. Kern Institute for the Transformation of Medical Education*.

Kelly, J. D. (2018). Forgiveness: A key resiliency builder. *Clinical Orthopaedics and Related Research*, *476*(2), 203–204. https://doi.org/10.1007/s11999.0000000000000024

Kleinman, A. (2015). Care: in search of a health agenda. *Lancet*, *386*(9990), 240–241. https://doi.org/10.1016/S0140-6736(15)61271-5

Kleinman, A. (2019). *The soul of care: The moral education of a husband and doctor*. Viking.

Kleinman, A. (2020). Varieties of experiences of care. *Perspectives in Biology and Medicine*, *63*(3), 458–465. https://doi.org/10.1353/pbm.2020.0033

Lawrence, E. C., Carvour, M. L., Camarata, C., Andarsio, E., & Rabow, M. W. (2020). Requiring the healer's art curriculum to promote professional identity formation among medical students. *Journal of Medical Humanities*, *41*(4), 531–541. https://doi.org/10.1007/s10912-020-09649-z

Lewin, L. O., McManamon, A., Stein, M. T. O., & Chen, D. T. (2019). Minding the form that transforms: Using Kegan's model of adult development to understand personal and professional identity formation in medicine. *Academic Medicine: Journal of the Association of American Medical Colleges*, *94*(9), 1299–1304. https://doi.org/10.1097/ACM.0000000000002741

Lönn, A., Weurlander, M., Seeberger, A., Hult, H., Thornberg, R., & Wernerson, A. (2023). The impact of emotionally challenging situations on medical students' professional identity formation. *Advances in Health Sciences Education: Theory and Practice*, 28(5), 1557–1578. https://doi.org/10.1007/s10459-023-10229-8

MacLeod, A. (2011). Caring, competence and professional identities in medical education. *Advances in Health Sciences Education: Theory and Practice*, 16(3), 375–394. https://doi.org/10.1007/s10459-010-9269-9

Matsui, T., Sato, M., Kato, Y., & Nishigori, H. (2019). Professional identity formation of female doctors in Japan—Gap between the married and unmarried. *BMC Medical Education*, 19(1), 55. https://doi.org/10.1186/s12909-019-1479-0

Mokhachane, M., George, A., Wyatt, T., Kuper, A., & Green-Thompson, L. (2023). Rethinking professional identity formation amidst protests and social upheaval: A journey in Africa. *Advances in Health Sciences Education: Theory and Practice*, 28(2), 427–452. https://doi.org/10.1007/s10459-022-10164-0

Monrouxe, L. V. (2010). Identity, identification and medical education: Why should we care? *Medical Education*, 44(1), 40–49. https://doi.org/10.1111/j.1365-2923.2009.03440.x

Morgan, A., Moore, J., & Duff, A. (2019). Guide the way: Tutored reflection facilitates professional identity formation. *Medical Teacher*, 41(2), 235–236. https://doi.org/10.1080/0142159X.2018.1515478

Mount, G. R., Kahlke, R., Melton, J., & Varpio, L. (2022). A critical review of professional identity formation interventions in medical education. *Academic Medicine: Journal of the Association of American Medical Colleges*, 97(11S), S96–S106. https://doi.org/10.1097/ACM.0000000000004904

Noddings, N. (1984). *Caring: A feminine approach to ethics and moral education.* University of California Press.

Nothnagle, M., Reis, S., Goldman, R. E., & Anandarajah, G. (2014). Fostering professional formation in residency: Development and evaluation of the "forum" seminar series. *Teaching and Learning in Medicine*, 26(3), 230–238. https://doi.org/10.1080/10401334.2014.910124

Ranasinghe, P. D., & Zhou, A. (2023). Women physicians and the COVID-19 pandemic: Gender-based impacts and potential interventions. *Annals of Medicine*, 55(1), 319–324. https://doi.org/10.1080/07853890.2022.2164046

Rees, C. E., & Monrouxe, L. V. (2018). Who are you and who do you want to be? Key considerations in developing professional identities in medicine. *Medical Journal of Australia*, 209(5), 202–203. https://doi.org/10.5694/mja18.00118

Rees, C. E., Kent, F., & Crampton, P. E. S. (2019). Student and clinician identities: How are identities constructed in interprofessional narratives? *Medical Education*, 53(8), 808–823. https://doi.org/10.1111/medu.13886

Sarraf-Yazdi, S., Goh, S., & Krishna, L. (2024). Conceptualizing professional identity formation in medicine. *Academic Medicine: Journal of the Association of American Medical Colleges*, 99(3), 343. https://doi.org/10.1097/ACM.0000000000005559

Shubkin, C. D., Garrett, J. R., & Lantos, J. D. (2018). When residents let conscience be their guide: Professional development and educational opportunity. *Academic Pediatrics*, 18(3), 239–242. https://doi.org/10.1016/j.acap.2017.12.003

Slotnick, H. B., & Hilton, S. R. (2006). Proto-professionalism and the dissecting laboratory. *Clinical Anatomy*, 19(5), 429–436. https://doi.org/10.1002/ca.20311

Sternszus, R., Slattery, N. K., Cruess, R. L., Cate, O. T., Hamstra, S. J., & Steinert, Y. (2023). Contradictions and opportunities: Reconciling professional identity formation and competency-based medical education. *Perspectives on Medical Education*, 12(1), 507–516. https://doi.org/10.5334/pme.1027

Tagawa, M. (2019). Development of a scale to evaluate medical professional identity formation. *BMC Medical Education*, 19(1), 63. https://doi.org/10.1186/s12909-019-1499-9

Trevino, R., & Poitevien, P. (2021). Professional identity formation for underrepresented in medicine learners. *Current Problems in Pediatric and Adolescent Health Care*, 51(10), 101091. https://doi.org/10.1016/j.cppeds.2021.101091

Tronto, J. C. (1993). *Moral boundaries: A political argument for an ethic of care*. Routledge. https://doi.org/10.4324/9781003070672

Veen, M., & de la Croix, A. (2023). How to grow a professional identity: Philosophical gardening in the field of medical education. *Perspectives on Medical Education*, 12(1), 12–19. https://doi.org/10.5334/pme.367

Wald, H. S., White, J., Reis, S. P., Esquibel, A. Y., & Anthony, D. (2019). Grappling with complexity: Medical students' reflective writings about challenging patient encounters as a window into professional identity formation. *Medical Teacher*, 41(2), 152–160. https://doi.org/10.1080/0142159X.2018.1475727

Webster-Wright, A. (2009). Reframing professional development through understanding authentic professional learning. *Review of Educational Research*, 79(2), 702–739. https://doi.org/10.3102/0034654308330970

Weston, W. W. (2005). Patient-centered medicine: A guide to the biopsychosocial model. *Families, Systems, & Health*, 23(4), 387–392. https://doi.org/10.1037/1091-7527.23.4.387

Wyatt, T. R., Balmer, D., Rockich-Winston, N., Chow, C. J., Richards, J., & Zaidi, Z. (2021). 'Whispers and shadows': A critical review of the professional identity literature with respect to minority physicians. *Medical Education*, 55, 148–158. https://doi.org/10.1111/medu.14295

Yiu, S., Yeung, M., Cheung, W. J., & Frank, J. R. (2023). Stress and conflict from tacit culture forges professional identity in newly graduated independent physicians. *Advances in Health Sciences Education: Theory and Practice*, 28(3), 847–870. https://doi.org/10.1007/s10459-022-10173-z

Yu, C., Liu, Q., Wang, W., Xie, A., & Liu, J. (2022). Professional identity of 0.24 million medical students in China before and during the COVID-19 pandemic: Three waves of national cross-sectional studies. *Frontiers in Public Health*, 10, 868914. https://doi.org/10.3389/fpubh.2022.868914

CHAPTER 10

Discussion

....

The art, science, and lived experience of becoming and being a physician compose the doctor's life cycle (DLC). As veterans of 46 and 40 years in family medicine, and 37 years in internal medicine, and as clinicians and medical educators in three distinct areas of the globe, we have each been pondering this mystery for decades. We have summoned the work of every scholar and writer we could get our hands on and reflected deeply upon our own maturational trajectory. What have we learned?

We have witnessed the emergence of the professional identity formation (PIF) construct, a theoretical framework comprehensive enough to bring together a vast array of previously disparate perspectives on the topic. With its link to professionalism and ethics, the PIF framework has captured the imagination of many scholars of professional education. A flurry of papers and books lends a solid theoretical and fair descriptive basis to the construct. Programs have adopted this approach and include curricula that are built around this organizing principle.[1,2]

1   Knox, A. B. (1977). *Adult development and learning: A handbook on individual growth and competence in the adult years.* Jossey-Bass.

2   Jayarathne, S. W., & Schuwirth, L. (2022). Exploring unlearning in the process of professional identity formation (PIF). *Asia Pacific Scholar,* 7(1), 106–108. https://doi.org/10.29060/TAPS.2022-7-1/PV2532

DOI: 10.1201/9781003507529-11

Yet, empirical data supporting the performance of this paradigm are lagging (Isaacson).[3]

Two concerns have emerged. First, the fact that most of the described categories, especially the more developed and updated ones, are heavily invested in the formative years of basic and graduate medical education (from medical school to the end of residency and perhaps fellowship), leaving the majority of a DLC—the practice years and transition to retirement and beyond—with little scholarly attention. Second, while it is clear that gender, ethnic, and racial diversity; external adverse events such as the coronavirus pandemic and war; and other societal changes have a decisive impact on the DLC, PIF is often viewed as homogeneous and unchanging over broad swaths of time.

THE BLIND SAGES AND THE ELEPHANT

It is very tempting to try to juggle stages and levels from different models into a synthetic view, but this is an exercise in mixing apples and oranges. The newer approaches clearly move away from a linear, though complicated, developmental model to a complex, dynamic, and constantly negotiated understanding. Separating the stages of PIF or other categories from their paradigmatic origin may result in losing much of their meaning. Many models, many lenses through which to peek at the elephant (the one from the fable with the six blind sages),[4] and many metaphors were identified. Multiple theories inform the categories and models, including complexity theory,[5] cognitive apprenticeship,[6] situated

---

3   Isaacson, J. H., Ziring, D., Hafferty, F., Kalet, A., Littleton, D., & Frankel, R. M. (2021). In search of medical professionalism research: Preliminary results from a review of widely read medical journals. The Permanente Journal, 25. https://doi.org/10.7812/TPP/20.223

4   *The parable of the blind sages and the elephant, in a nutshell*: Six blind sages endeavor to accurately describe an elephant, but each is only able to describe the part he is touching (ears, tusks, tail, and so on), thereby failing to perceive the entire elephant, or "the whole picture."

5   Long, K. M., McDermott, F., & Meadows, G. N. (2018). Being pragmatic about healthcare complexity: Our experiences applying complexity theory and pragmatism to health services research. *BMC Medicine*, 16(1), 94. https://doi.org/10.1186/s12916-018-1087-6

6   Merritt, C., Daniel, M., Munzer, B. W., Nocera, M., Ross, J. C., & Santen, S. A. (2018). A cognitive apprenticeship-based faculty development intervention for emergency medicine educators. *Western Journal of Emergency Medicine*, 19(1), 198–204. https://doi.org/10.5811/westjem.2017.11.36429

learning, communities of practice, figured worlds,[7] socialization theory, the Personality and Social Structure Perspective (PSSP), cultural–historical activity theory (CHAT),[8] and, finally, rites of passage and liminality.

COMPLEXITY AND THE DOCTOR'S LIFE CYCLE

Complexity theory may be helpful as an organizing paradigm for the DLC. Here we attempt a brief introduction to the theory for the reader encountering complexity in medical education for the first time. **Mennin**[9] describes complexity science as follows:

> A collection of concepts and principles for the study of open systems that have nonlinear, dynamical, self-organizing and emergent properties. Complexity science is the study of the dynamics of patterns and relationships rather than objects and substance in systems that are open and far from equilibrium. Complexity science focuses on processes and interactions of local agents that result in the emergence of new patterns.

> A system composed of a large number of components that can be described completely based on its individual constituents is complicated. Computers, jet planes and rocket ships are complicated. A system composed of many diverse components is complex if the interactions among the components are such that the system as a whole cannot be understood by analysing its components.

PIF and medical education are increasingly recognized as complex adaptive systems and as such are not amenable to analysis through the mere understanding of their components.

The complexity of the DLC and PIF entails nonlinearity, self-organization, and emergent properties. Theoretically, it demands a multidimensional stance, and, practically, the PIF facilitator is invited to seek experiences, feedback, and reflection to provide conditions conducive to

7   Cantillon, P., De Grave, W., & Dornan, T. (2022). The social construction of teacher and learner identities in medicine and surgery. *Medical Education*, 56(6), 614–624. https://doi.org/10.1111/medu.14727

8   Elmberger, A., Björck, E., Liljedahl, M., Nieminen, J., & Bolander Laksov, K. (2019). Contradictions in clinical teachers' engagement in educational development: An activity theory analysis. *Advances in Health Sciences Education: Theory and Practice*, 24(1), 125–140. https://doi.org/10.1007/s10459-018-9853-y

9   Mennin, S. (2010). Complexity and health professions education: A basic glossary. *Journal of Evaluation in Clinical Practice*, 16, 838–840. https://doi.org/10.1111/j.1365-2753.2010.01503.x

self-organization and emergence. A special place is reserved for work at the edge of chaos (the zone of proximal development [ZPD]) through the constructs of liminality and the "crucible of learning" (described later in this chapter), which seem to be operating in the developmental and relational space where PIF is shaped and transformation may emerge.

METAPHORS OF THE DOCTOR'S LIFE CYCLE

The second lens that emerged as helpful is that of metaphors. Three metaphors stood out while immersing ourselves as described. The first, Marcus's **baking metaphor**, describes continuous kneading of dough that is the emergent practitioner's inner life, subsequently in need of the furnace's heat to produce sustaining bread. Thus, metaphorically, one is continuously forming on the professional journey in two stages: the first preparatory (kneading dough) and the second transformative (baking).

The second metaphor is the **bridge metaphor**, mentioned in Chapter 9 in conjunction with Kegan's model and expanded upon by **Schei** et al. and **Groot** et al. with the ZPD construct, and by Gordon et al. with liminality. Here, the developing practitioner is no longer fully preoccupied with the identity she is leaving behind yet is still not fully assuming the emerging identity. Thus, she is in an in-between "split" stance and engaged in identity work.

The third metaphor, introduced by Bleakley[10] based on writing by the poet **Wallace Stevens**, is **Force versus Presence**. He argues:

> Modern medicine has been shaped historically by the combative metaphor of a "war against disease," turning medicine into a quasi-militaristic culture fond of hierarchy. This is supplemented by the metaphor of the "body as machine," reducing the complex and unpredictable body to a linear, if complicated, apparatus. The two metaphors align medicine … [as] masculine, heroic, and controlling in character. In an era in which medicine is feminising and expected to be patient-centred, collaborative (inter-professional) and transparent to the public as a democratic gesture … this continuing dominance of Force over Presence matters because it is a style running counter to the collaborative, team-based medicine needed for high levels of patient safety. Medicine will authentically democratise only as new, pacific shaping metaphors emerge, those

10 Bleakley, A. (2017). Force and presence in the world of medicine. *Healthcare*, *5*(3), 58. https://doi.org/10.3390/healthcare5030058

of "Presence," such as "hospitality." Hospitals can once again become places of hospitality.

Force over Presence can also come from external influences and further expand the moral ideal-moral reality gap. Ideologies, regimes, state regulations, economics, wars, pandemics, planetary health, and racism are among the structural forces that shape the becoming, being, and practice of physicians across the globe. While the literature is mostly dominated by the Western-educated and practicing physician, where are the experiences of a physician in eastern Ukraine, rural India, Gaza, or remote regions of Somalia acknowledged?

This third metaphor ties together constructs that we have identified repeatedly: power and abuse of power (bias, discrimination, mistreatment), care versus justice, and care versus competence. It also points to how Presence and hospitality may be nurtured, and how medicine ripples with woundedness, bias, and the pandemic, the recent additional concerns.

INSIGHTS

Through this complex and metaphorical lens, we now segue to a set of insights that serve as a summary of our inquiry into the DLC.

1. From stages to complexity, ontology before epistemology. A body of knowledge about the DLC consisting of reasonable theoretical and fair descriptive underpinnings, with an emergent empirical component, exists. PIF is the most useful paradigm in this realm because it synthesizes recurrent themes, embraces sophisticated ideas that have emerged from the relevant discourses, and, as a developmental theory, provides a framework for the observed stages and transitions in a DLC. However, critics of professional development stage models emphasize the great variation in individual trajectories not accounted for in unified developmental theories. They emphasize the "who" of becoming a professional above and beyond what she knows and knows how to do as foundational to professional identity. These critics and others plead for a more complex and nuanced view, a realization that multiple identities are at work, with embodied primordial ones such as gender, ethnicity, and culture always present. All these views are likely to be useful lenses on the DLC. We believe that most of us recognize a substantial shared identity as doctors, while at the same time being profoundly and uniquely our own selves.

In any individual context, social influences exert a constant impact as our professional identities emerge. Reductionist, linear models fail to capture the complexity of this emergence. Ontology (lived experience) likely does and probably takes precedence over epistemology (conceptual clarity), as the opening narratives in this book show. A complex view of professional formation offers a shift from perceiving this process merely as an individual's cumulative gaining of knowledge and skills to addressing underlying individual, structural, and environmental factors that shape social actors and actions. This view "seeks to recast social actors, social structures, and environmental factors as interactive, adaptive, and interdependent."[11]

Present-day health professionals operate in "complex adaptive health systems in an environment of volatility, uncertainty, complexity, and ambiguity [that] likely requires individuals who have begun to develop *self-transforming* minds."[12] This self-transforming mind is the ultimate or most mature developmental stage of PIF according to Kegan, along with the master expertise stage, master adaptive learning, and phronesis. Coupling the intrapsychic with both socialization and context, complexity theory introduces the useful constructs of self-organization, paradox, edge of chaos, emergence, the benefit of instability, turbulence, and minimizing structure. Integrating complexity theory into our present understanding of PIF expands our understanding of the DLC. Additionally, both established and emergent standalone constructs in medical education, such as moral development, moral injury, power and control, practical wisdom (phronesis), rites of passage, intuition, courage, compassion and wisdom, "difficult" patients as the "moral stress test," virtue and character, caregiving, embodiment, conscience, risk of abuse of power, ethos of imperfection, embodied understanding of practice versus progression of skill, and identity complexity can all find a place in the complex notion of PIF. Each constitutes an aspect of this tapestry that we are attempting to integrate. Each can be perceived as the elephant if we position ourselves as one of the six blind sages. The complexity lens, along with ontology (the metaphors and narratives), enables viewing the whole elephant.

---

11 Hafferty, F. W., & Levinson, D. (2008). Moving beyond nostalgia and motives: Towards a complexity science view of medical professionalism. *Perspectives in Biology and Medicine*, 51(4), 599–615. https://doi.org/10.1353/pbm.0.0044

12 Lewin, L. O., McManamon, A., Stein, M. T. O., & Chen, D. T. (2019). Minding the form that transforms: Using Kegan's model of adult development to understand personal and professional identity formation in medicine. *Academic Medicine: Journal of the Association of American Medical Colleges*, 94(9), 1299–1304. https://doi.org/10.1097/ACM.0000000000002741

2. Moral development as an example. A striking example of this emergent understanding of the DLC is the analysis of category 4, moral and character development, which demonstrates the anomalies in the standard, accepted approach. Thus, principled ethics, as useful as it may be, is inadequate in addressing the day-to-day needs of a practitioner. The moral experience–moral ideal gap, the narrative nature of moral experience, the understanding that moral distress and injury are prevalent, the constant threat of abuse of power, and the shift from the dominant discourse of competence to one of presence have not yet found their way sufficiently into the current moral development discourse—but they should.

This insight is synergistic and resonates with the newer categories of remediation, bias, and the pandemic (categories 6–8). It calls for us to complexify our views and for a radical shift in bioethics pedagogy to incorporate vulnerability, failures, errors, the need for remediation, and conscious awareness of the ZPD. This view is useful for medical education, but particularly for the moral education of the physician which, practically speaking, needs to exit the lecture hall and become integrated with practice. Interactive, real-life pedagogies whereby lived moral experiences are processed both in their conceptual and experiential dimensions are needed. Attention is thus shifted from the informative to the formative and transformative levels. The result is a transformed moral education of the health practitioner, enabling the maximization of her full developmental moral potential and consequently the transformation of the doctor's ethical practice.

3. The "crucible of learning" or "the crucible of optional development" (or lack thereof); polarities as the yin and yang of development. Throughout this inquiry, recurring themes that identify polarities and paradoxes, as well as core conflicts and core transitions with a binary outcome, are described. These include empathy versus emotional disengagement, doing and being, tolerance of uncertainty versus a search for evidence, vulnerability versus an illusion of invulnerability (and its price), boundary maintenance versus boundary crossing, competence and care discourses, burnout and resilience, change and stability, emotions versus cognition, tolerance for uncertainty versus taming of hubris, active versus passive, helplessness versus problem solving, moral ideal and moral experience, explicit and implicit, hidden and formal curriculum, formation versus deformation, discrimination and inclusion (gender and race), and diversity and xenophobia. This is just a partial list of the many tensions at play in the DLC.

How do these polarities play out over the developmental journey? As mentioned, Frank describes physician narratives and classifies them into chaos, triumph, and quest stories. The mindful practitioner may transcend failure and success and embark on a quest where the dualities are replaced by expansion of the comfort zone. Polarities are the yin and yang of development, challenging the evolving practitioner to hang in there so that neither takes over and a breakthrough, transition, or learning may be achieved, while containing the challenge of polarity and accepting it as a source of further development.

Thus, a landscape of ever-present polarities, conflicts, and tasks is the territory of the practitioner's lifelong journey. Obviously, it is rare that any one physician faces all these aspects. Should more be done to make the implicit yin and yang of development explicit? This is where reflection, mindfulness training, reflective writing, narrative medicine, and related pedagogies become useful, fostering recovery, remoralization, and potential growth.

Most of the literature conveys a sense of achievement (of expertise, mature morality, and ideal identity), while failures are discussed mostly under the heading of errors or "impaired physician." Yet, each doctor's life cycle contains crises, regressions, and arrests in development. This realization is addressed sparingly under the "formation versus deformation" heading, as well as in the burnout and impaired physician discourses. This splitting diverts attention from the ubiquitous presence of these events. Failures and errors can produce learning and development: a phased recovery process is described, and empirical data on the utility and outcomes of remediation are available. Moreover, this inquiry demonstrates that vulnerability is practically ever-present, along with a frequent sense of helplessness. When embraced, these may be conditions necessary for development, as painful and challenging as it may be. Such situations are not only about dealing with burnout or fostering resilience in the face of professional and personal adversity, but about what simulation has taught us: failure (if at all possible, in an unpunishing milieu such as simulation) may be a mighty development stimulus.

Based on this inquiry, a new construct has emerged. The idea of the **crucible of learning** is as follows: when faced with trials such as cognitive dissonance, uncertainty, failure, compassion fatigue, and demoralization, a learning and growth crucible may become available. By accepting these situations—along with potential accompanying feelings of helplessness, vulnerability, and shame, as well as the need for apology and forgiveness of oneself and others—and seeking to transcend them, the practitioner may ultimately increase her comfort zone and further expand her ZPD. Easier said than done. In the literature, emerging pedagogies support resilience and conditioning of health professionals to embrace low moments as painful but also as potential sources of growth.[13] Continuous Medical Education (CME), for example, may translate into a needs-based CME paradigm[14] that also addresses errors, failures, and emotional and metacognitive needs as legitimate CME and continuous professional development goals.

Learning, be it informative, formative, or transformative, happens in many ways. First, the simple accumulation of knowledge, skills, understanding, and competencies is how learning to become a physician is classically described and experienced, what Weston calls "gaining medical knowledge and technical competence in dealing with disease."[15] It is possible, through simulation, that the emotional and practical price of this learning may be minimized. This is what Kegan calls the informative level, the one that begets experts.

A second process, "becoming" a professional, a formation, stems from additional identity work as well as working through errors, failures, and crises. However, when a patient experiences an adverse outcome, the pain of the physician herself may become excruciating, even deadly. Stages of recovery and restitution have been described (Chapter 6). The concept of formation is gaining momentum in current medical education and, as described by Kegan, it begets professionals.

The third learning stage, learning to heal, transformative this time (Kegan again), ripples with the crucible of learning and can be described as follows: when a learner encounters a learning need and attempts to address it, she may need to move to the edges of her comfort zone (the ZPD—intellectually, procedurally, emotionally, or even existentially). In this realm of being, vulnerability and a sense of helplessness necessarily prevail. However, having experienced that these painful conditions are the ones that beget the most valuable lessons and enable transformation, the learner yields to them and immerses herself in the difficulty and discomfort. Here, stretching one's comfort zone and pushing hard at

13 Molloy, E., & Bearman, M. (2019). Embracing the tension between vulnerability and credibility: 'Intellectual candour' in health professions education. *Medical Education*, *53*(1), 32–41. https://doi.org/10.1111/medu.13649

14 Norman, G. R., Shannon, S. I., & Marrin, M. L. (2004). The need for needs assessment in continuing medical education. *BMJ Clinical Research*, *328*(7446), 999–1001. https://doi.org/10.1136/bmj.328.7446.999

15 Weston, W. W., Brown, J. B. (2024). Becoming a physician: The human experience of medical education. In Stewart, M., Brown, J. B., Weston, W. W., Freeman, T. R., Ryan, B. L., McWilliam, C. L., and McWhinney, I. R. (eds). Patient-centered medicine: Transforming the clinical method (4th ed). CRC Press.

boundaries enables development. If ignored or failed, growth is stunted: the growth curve of either expertise or PIF flattens or starts to decline (see Chapter 9, Figure 9.1). This is when, without intervention, development is replaced by disability, arrests, and possible decline. This learning crucible presents itself in many ways. Its prevalence is not known, and while it is intellectually and experientially attractive, it needs further description and validation.

While the crucible of learning has been described here as facilitating transformative learning, it may also apply to the informative and formative levels. The following are some examples:

a. **Patient care.** Moments of uncertainty, ambivalence, and lack of clarity are common, and summon the practitioner to "hang in there." In such moments, full engagement of the self, the ventriloquist (speaking for the patient who has no words for their suffering), and the witness (being there, to validate and acknowledge the patient's experience) functions of a practitioner may be instrumental, and metacognition may emerge. Thus, the crucible of learning may support clinical decision-making, especially in "stuck" and complex situations. Extrapolating from moral development, difficult patient care episodes are the "stress test" of PIF and clinical problem-solving.

b. **Teaching.** Coaching, mentoring, and role modeling, alongside welcoming challenging and "impossible" clinical, contextual, and relational situations, are called for. Debriefing and emotion processing may also be helpful for better navigation of this crucible. Aiming for formative and transformative learning should be adopted as recommended, with the facilitating pedagogies applied.[16]

c. **Learning.** Welcoming uncertainty, embracing chaos, respecting the learning gained from an adverse example ("learning by scar formation"[17]), attending and developing as mindful practitioners, utilizing narrative and reflection, and sharing in peer groups and communities of practice are some of the habits of mind that support learning in the described "crucible."

d. **Curriculum development.** PIF and other identified constructs should be explicitly included in the medical education curriculum, including lifelong learning, adaptive expertise, moral development, and

---

16 Borrell-Carrió, F., Suchman, A. L., & Epstein, R. M. (2004). The biopsychosocial model 25 years later: Principles, practice, and scientific inquiry. *Annals of Family Medicine, 2*(6), 576–582. https://doi.org/10.1370/afm.245

17 Schuwirth, L. (2004). Learning by scar formation. *Medical Education, 38*(8), 797–799. https://doi.org/10.1111/j.1365-2929.2004.01906.x

narrative competence. The curriculum needs to deal with ensuring emotional health, work–home balance, resilience, and identity work. It needs to explicitly focus on instructional methods and content that transcend informative curricula toward formative and transformative ones. Special attention needs to be given to addressing transitions.

e. **Assessment.** Measures that monitor development are needed. Emotion-laden scenarios (in objective structured clinical examinations [OSCEs], for example) should supplement knowledge and procedural skills and incorporate emotional, communicative, and moral challenges. Assessment should adopt a developmental stance so that the proto-practitioner can be informed of her progress on the prescribed trajectory.[18]

f. **Transitions.** These should be paid special attention. Acknowledging vulnerability, helplessness, "failure," liminality, the practitioner's position on the "bridge," being "not fully baked," getting familiar with death and dying, seeking transcendence, and welcoming support in coping with transitions are relevant here. Respecting and celebrating emotions as well as efforts to build resilience by exposure to situations where cognition must be maximized and any emotions that divert attention and focus suspended (but subsequently processed)—such as difficult surgery or procedures, complex emergencies, disaster medicine, and pandemics—are all also helpful (as difficult as they may be) in supporting meaningful, developmentally oriented learning.

g. **External obstacles.** We need scholarship explicating the impact of both welcome and unwelcome difficulties on the DLC, and how to prepare practitioners to recognize their ZPD or create a crucible of learning in even the direst of circumstances. The ability to face extreme challenges with professional capabilities intact is likely to be highly individual yet learnable.

To meet the challenge of applying the crucible of learning, frameworks for individual learning need to be complemented by a sophisticated understanding of social learning, such as in the learning community theory. The evolving individual practitioner is on a dynamic lifelong journey in her learning community. The critical influences of the setting and

---

18 Sawatsky, A. P., O'Brien, B. C., & Hafferty, F. W. (2022). Autonomy and developing physicians: Reimagining supervision using self-determination theory. *Medical Education*, 56(1), 56–63. https://doi.org/10.1111/medu.14580

community in which the DLC takes place are of utmost significance and need to be further researched and deciphered.

4. A wake-up call: structural disadvantages with regard to gender, race, ethnicity, and other core identities, and related bias, discrimination, and mistreatment. The added developmental and practical stressors that gender, race, and additional stigmatized identities bring to the DLC, as compared to the "normative" practitioner, are described and acknowledged. Despite progress in diversifying the profession, and because of that progress, a great deal must still be addressed to ensure that all practitioners can develop and thrive over a lifetime of practice. While policies and practices that support a more diverse physician workforce have been proposed, implementation is inconsistent and the outcomes unclear.[19]

In conducting this inquiry, we were shaken by the persistence of evidence displaying how power, racism, and misogyny continue to exert an oppressive and disabling impact on physician formation. Presented here are the components of this realization extracted from the literature: Medicine is prone to abuse of power, both toward patients and within the profession. Power is intimately related to identity formation, as identity is permeated with multiple forms of power. One manifestation of the misuse of power in medicine is the paucity of attention to gender, race, and other marginalized identities. As a result, study of the DLC and PIF is likely biased and in need of reexamination and soul-searching reform in its conduct around issues of power, gender, race, bias, and abuse.

Furthermore, as Bleakley notes, "women are in the majority in terms of entry to medical schools worldwide and will soon represent the majority of working doctors. This has been termed the 'feminising' of medicine."[20] As such, it may be time to reflect on the implications of this reality beyond the sheer composition of the medical workforce. Again, Bleakley stands out by proclaiming:

> In medical education, such gender issues tend to be restricted to discussions of demographic changes and structural inequalities based on a biological reading of gender. However, in contemporary social sciences, gender theory has moved beyond both biology and demography to

---

19 Elfaki, L. A., Groenewoud, R., Nwakoby, A., Zubair, A., Verma, R., & Yanagawa, B. (2024). 2023 update on equity, diversity, and inclusion in Canadian cardiac surgery. *Current Opinion in Cardiology*, 39(1), 68–71. https://doi.org/10.1097/HCO .0000000000001101

20 Bleakley, A. (2013). Gender matters in medical education. *Medical Education*, 47(1), 59–70. https://doi.org/10.1111/j.1365-2923.2012.04351.x

include cultural issues of gendered ways of thinking. Can contemporary feminist thought drawn from the social sciences help medical educators to widen their appreciation and understanding of the feminising of medicine?

This discussion would be incomplete without once again acknowledging the pandemic. The crisis, the death toll, the profound transformation of life and healthcare, the enormous ethical issues, and the moral, psychological, and physical distress are compelling a review of beliefs, practices, and mindsets. The pandemic disproportionately affected vulnerable populations and created an unequal burden for disenfranchised provider groups such as women and minorities.

Thus, the pandemic provided an alarming wake-up call. It extensively curtailed learners' exposure to patients for physical examinations and clinical care and had a profound influence on both medical student and postgraduate trajectories. How will the identities of physicians who were involved, both in the early and late phases of their trajectories, be molded by COVID-19? The answer is still unknown. Consequently, humanity as well as health professionals are thrust into a liminal phase. One enduring lesson is the imperative of paying attention to learner and practitioner wellbeing.

The life cycle paradigm is informed by the complex nature of competence, role, and identity. It is composed of a dynamic series of learning moments and transitions, whether through failure, error, and helplessness, or through triumph and a sense of achievement, mindful quest, skill and competency acquisition, or obligatory liminality. Medical education needs to integrate this vision and perspective into its most progressive paradigms and discourse, and operationalize them in curricula, teaching methods, assessment, and an ethos of professional identity formation monitoring that seeks the best balance of learner and practitioner wellbeing and the maximization of potential.

CONCLUSIONS

1. The goals of medical education require a fresh, synergistic, and complex overhaul of physician formation. PIF and DLC discourses should aim to encourage formative and transformative learning.
2. Professional discourse on the DLC is also entering a new stage, with identity, role, power, location, and liminality identified as necessary constructs complementary to the competence and care discourses.
3. The core identities discourse is currently highlighting gender, race,

ethnicity, special needs and disability, and sexual orientation. Attention to these and their unfolding in the DLC is warranted. Implementation of policies intended to address diversity, inclusion, and structural competence should continue to be questioned and challenged to protect against unintended negative consequences and ensure that the discourse is factually rigorous, respectful, civil, and unbiased. The goal of inclusion should be accountable, excellent practice that serves the needs of our patients and communities.

4. It is time to better understand physician life cycle transitions and crises, as well as breakthroughs and nodal points or nuanced stages of development and transition, and their associated identity work. Liminality may be a useful construct for guiding transition work. During transitions, trainees or practitioners are liminars and are invited to "actively occupy liminality" to maximize the transitions' success. Organizations and systems should recognize and support high-stakes transitions. Studying the role of and influences on socializing factors (informed also by complexity science, if possible) using natural experiments—such as new medical schools, shifts in postgraduate training, new models of continuous professional development, continuous medical education, remediation, and adversarial contexts—can help optimize physician development and flourishing.

5. Transformation-seeking instructional methods that address power, role, care, and identity, and are informed by the constructs and insights described in this book, should be developed and evaluated.

6. We need measurements and evaluations of roles and identities, lifespan development, PIF, and more to study and inform our understanding and enhancement of physicianhood.

7. Engaging with sister disciplines that are also immersed in similar scholarly inquiry can advance the emerging dialogue on the DLC. Gathering all the relevant scholars will help further this work.

8. Exploring the facilitators of expertise and mastery formation in the periods beyond becoming a board-certified specialist will provide further elucidation. This exploration is likely to include deliberate practice, the master adaptive learner approach, and the quest for peak performance and the acquisition of phronesis, a developmental framework that highlights the location of a ZPD. Its aim should be to maximize physician potential.

9. We hope for a breakthrough, as described, in the scholarly pursuit of moral and character development in healthcare. This inquiry needs to extend beyond virtue ethics and current definitions of professionalism to include explorations of the potential for the abuse of

power, the actual misuse of power, and its interaction with identity formation. Emphasis should be placed on equity and the differential experiences of those from disenfranchised groups.

10. The notion of the crucible of learning and development needs to be further investigated and explored in all relevant educational and career components.

CLOSING THOUGHTS

The physician's life cycle is a reality in search of better understanding. To this end, progress is made with the integration of constructs such as complexity, master adaptive learning, PIF, and descriptions of identity work, especially during life transitions. A crucible of learning—a growth development node that also incorporates liminality—emerges in most categories. It is another take on the ZPD, where a learner pushes the limits of her comfort zone, choosing to be a liminar and facing vulnerability, uncertainty, and unease in order to grow and expand into a zone of proximal discovery. The metaphors of baking, bridge-crossing, and presence help communicate a nuanced understanding of this growth trajectory.

These constructs lend themselves to the operationalization of curricula, pedagogies, and assessment that can facilitate the journey and need to be incorporated into medical education. While there is no single unifying model that integrates all the myriad approaches and insights, this investigation advances the DLC from the "blind sages and the elephant" stage to a limited number of interrelated components that start to form a plausible model around the PIF framework while also transcending it. Identified blind spots concern inequity, discrimination, mistreatment, and lack of attention to the experiences of women, ethnic minorities, and marginalized identities in the DLC, as well as the adverse challenges posed by external forces such as war, politics, and economics. The aforementioned conclusions are routes that may draw us nearer to a conceptual framework with the power to enhance effective education, mentoring, and a coherent approach for both professional identity formation and its multiple transitions.

At the conclusion of this quest, a clearer view of the issue at hand is available, also enabled by the synergistic progress of recent work. The integrative emergent constructs include a more nuanced developmental stage model and an integration of adult learning with the expertise categories into the master adaptive learner concept, both within the informative–formative–transformative paradigm incorporating and situating

PIF. Moral development is singled out as a paradigm in need of revision post-COVID-19, with a roadmap on how to achieve it, while narrative and reflection are upheld as essential for the transition to the formative and transformative levels. In addition, the downside (albeit essential) of development is brought into focus. Failures, errors, and developmental arrests, as well as structural barriers (external adverse circumstances) and the influences of discrimination, abuse, and mistreatment, are compounded by wars, racism, and climate change and constitute formidable challenges at times.

The evolving practitioner struggles first and foremost with her competence on the informative level. Once committed to quality assurance and lifelong learning (hopefully self-regulated), she may or may not succeed at this level. If she does not or cannot, she will find herself struggling, mostly on autopilot (possibly with routine expertise), and will unfortunately fall short of her potential. An unknown portion of physicians worldwide progress to the next, formative level. Invested in their PIF, introspective, and reflective, they seek and reach not only expertise but also phronesis and mastery. They must be, at least tacitly, aficionados of the crucible of learning, ZPD, and liminality. Through liminality, identity, and developmental work, they make their way into mature physicianhood. A further minority will progress, albeit through trials and tribulations, to the transformative level and achieve fuller actualization of their potential to become master adaptive learners, phronetic, and "enlightened change agents."[21]

In each step of the journey, physicians belong to communities of practice that go through a developmental journey of their own with a collective ZPD and collective expertise, as well as optional collective formative and transformative levels. On a larger level, physicians are also part of a complex healthcare system with both uplifting and demoralizing aspects. This very complex, nonlinear system defies simplification and reductionism. It demands submission to the polarized nature of the different process components, obligatory vulnerability, and immersion in liminality and transitions in order to hopefully expand. It is too often

---

21 Frenk, J., Chen, L., Bhutta, Z. A., Cohen, J., Crisp, N., Evans, T., Fineberg, H., Garcia, P., Ke, Y., Kelley, P., Kistnasamy, B., Meleis, A., Naylor, D., Pablos-Mendez, A., Reddy, S., Scrimshaw, S., Sepulveda, J., Serwadda, D., & Zurayk, H. (2010). Health professionals for a new century: Transforming education to strengthen health systems in an interdependent world. *The Lancet, 376*(9756), 1923–1958. https://doi.org/10.1016/S0140-6736(10)61854-5

growth by scar formation. Becoming and being a physician is potentially the most exhilarating and terrible journey all at the same time.

We do hope that this book will find echoes in the professional discourse and launch further scholarly and practical conversations that may result in additional understanding and application. One dimension that we hardly touched is the political one: medicine is political, and its delivery is always shaped by local and global general and professional politics. COVID-19 was a somber reminder of this fact, exposing the enormous gaps between rich and poor, white and people of color, east and west, north and south, capitalists and socialists. Bleakley stands out as a scholar who studies this angle relentlessly. We have quoted him several times but refrained from a full investigation of this aspect. We must recognize our limitations, and this is one.

The stories opening each of the preceding chapters in this book connect the conceptual inquiry to physicians' lived experience. They are predominantly the fruits of our (the authors') lived experience. As practitioners, we have a healthy suspicion of highbrow theoreticians. Lived experience is messier than depictions in scholarly accounts, even when they address messy recesses. The transformation of a layperson into a physician, and even more so into one who is mature and as fully developed as possible, remains a mystery. The tension between scholarship, narratives, and lived experience is the ultimate crucible of learning in which we are now immersed and invite you to join.

As veteran physicians, we have experienced these strands in each of our own journeys. We embody, at the same time, failures and peak performance, arrests and breakthroughs, demoralization and remoralization, smooth sailing, and liminality. Facing the late stages of our professional life cycle, we are wrapping up the active clinical practice phase and transitioning to a stage where we can reflect on a rich and fulfilling life of doctoring. Returning to the Introduction, we do not feel as Sassall does that our work as physicians justifies our lives, but it has certainly made us fortunate and humble. We have served as both healers and educators. In this reflection on what others have said about the journey, we have had the privilege to be "students of human nature and moral wisdom." We embarked on this study to both make sense of the education we have received and given, and hopefully provide guidance to those who seek to take this journey after us. We look forward to the continued quests of our colleagues and readers and look forward to your insights.

REFERENCES

Bleakley, A. (2013). Gender matters in medical education. *Medical Education*, *47*(1), 59–70. https://doi.org/10.1111/j.1365-2923.2012.04351.x

Borrell-Carrió, F., Suchman, A. L., & Epstein, R. M. (2004). The biopsychosocial model 25 years later: Principles, practice, and scientific inquiry. *Annals of Family Medicine*, *2*(6), 576–582. https://doi.org/10.1370/afm.245

Cantillon, P., De Grave, W., & Dornan, T. (2022). The social construction of teacher and learner identities in medicine and surgery. *Medical Education*, *56*(6), 614–624. https://doi.org/10.1111/medu.14727

Elfaki, L. A., Groenewoud, R., Nwakoby, A., Zubair, A., Verma, R., & Yanagawa, B. (2024). 2023 update on equity, diversity, and inclusion in Canadian cardiac surgery. *Current Opinion in Cardiology*, *39*(1), 68–71. https://doi.org/10.1097/HCO .0000000000001101

Elmberger, A., Björck, E., Liljedahl, M., Nieminen, J., & Bolander Laksov, K. (2019). Contradictions in clinical teachers' engagement in educational development: An activity theory analysis. *Advances in Health Sciences Education: Theory and Practice*, *24*(1), 125–140. https://doi.org/10.1007/s10459-018-9853-y

Frenk, J., Chen, L., Bhutta, Z. A., Cohen, J., Crisp, N., Evans, T., Fineberg, H., Garcia, P., Ke, Y., Kelley, P., Kistnasamy, B., Meleis, A., Naylor, D., Pablos-Mendez, A., Reddy, S., Scrimshaw, S., Sepulveda, J., Serwadda, D., & Zurayk, H. (2010). Health professionals for a new century: Transforming education to strengthen health systems in an interdependent world. *The Lancet*, *376*(9756), 1923–1958. https://doi. org/10.1016/S0140-6736(10)61854-5

Hafferty, F. W., & Levinson, D. (2008). Moving beyond nostalgia and motives: Towards a complexity science view of medical professionalism. *Perspectives in Biology and Medicine*, *51*(4), 599–615. https://doi.org/10.1353/pbm.0.0044

Isaacson, J. H., Ziring, D., Hafferty, F., Kalet, A., Littleton, D., & Frankel, R. M. (2021). In search of medical professionalism research: Preliminary results from a review of widely read medical journals. *The Permanente Journal*, *25*. https://doi.org/10.7812 /TPP/20.223

Jayarathne, S. W., & Schuwirth, L. (2022). Exploring unlearning in the process of professional identity formation (PIF). *Asia Pacific Scholar*, *7*(1), 106–108. https://doi .org/10.29060/TAPS.2022-7-1/PV2532

Knox, A. B. (1977). *Adult development and learning: A handbook on individual growth and competence in the adult years*. Jossey-Bass

Lewin, L. O., McManamon, A., Stein, M. T. O., & Chen, D. T. (2019). Minding the form that transforms: Using Kegan's model of adult development to understand personal and professional identity formation in medicine. *Academic Medicine: Journal of the Association of American Medical Colleges*, *94*(9), 1299–1304. https://doi. org/10.1097/ACM.0000000000002741

Long, K. M., McDermott, F., & Meadows, G. N. (2018). Being pragmatic about healthcare complexity: Our experiences applying complexity theory and pragmatism to health services research. *BMC Medicine*, *16*(1), 94. https://doi.org/10.1186/s12916-018 -1087-6

Mennin, S. (2010). Complexity and health professions education: A basic glossary. *Journal of Evaluation in Clinical Practice*, *16*, 838–840. https://doi.org/10.1111/j .1365-2753.2010.01503.x

Merritt, C., Daniel, M., Munzer, B. W., Nocera, M., Ross, J. C., & Santen, S. A. (2018). A cognitive apprenticeship-based faculty development intervention for emergency medicine educators. *Western Journal of Emergency Medicine*, *19*(1), 198–204. https://doi.org/10.5811/westjem.2017.11.36429

Molloy, E., & Bearman, M. (2019). Embracing the tension between vulnerability and credibility: 'Intellectual candour' in health professions education. *Medical Education*, 53(1), 32–41. https://doi.org/10.1111/medu.13649

Norman, G. R., Shannon, S. I., & Marrin, M. L. (2004). The need for needs assessment in continuing medical education. *BMJ Clinical Research*, 328(7446), 999–1001. https://doi.org/10.1136/bmj.328.7446.999

Sawatsky, A. P., O'Brien, B. C., & Hafferty, F. W. (2022). Autonomy and developing physicians: Reimagining supervision using self-determination theory. *Medical Education*, 56(1), 56–63. https://doi.org/10.1111/medu.14580

Schuwirth, L. (2004). Learning by scar formation. *Medical Education*, 38(8), 797–799. https://doi.org/10.1111/j.1365-2929.2004.01906.x

Weston, W. W., & Brown, J. B. (2024). Becoming a physician: The human experience of medical education. In Stewart, M., Brown, J. B., Weston, W. W., Freeman, T. R., Ryan, B. L., McWilliam, C. L., and McWhinney, I. R. (eds). Patient-centered medicine: Transforming the clinical method (4th ed). CRC Press.

Epilogue

Ronald M. Epstein, MD
Professor of Family Medicine, Oncology and Medicine (Palliative
Care); American Cancer Society Clinical Research Professor,
Co-Director; Center for Communication and Disparities Research,
University of Rochester Medical Center, Rochester, New York

George Orwell, known for his vividly dark dystopic portrayals of socio-political oppression in *1984* and *Animal Farm*, and for risking his life more than once to promote freedom, would come home and care for his roses. So the account goes, as passionate as he was about his work saving the world from tyranny, his strength came from individual relationships and aesthetic pursuits. In an inspiring recent article, Iona Heath and Victor Montori[1] propose that our individual "roses" are a vital part of our professional identities as physicians and can be a prescription for the growth and sustainability of intellectually and emotionally intense careers.

One of my "roses" is playing music. As an amateur musician, I find harmony, balance, and transcendence when I sit at the keyboard. The experience is as much in sensations—in my fingers and in my ears—as it is in emotions. Music is dizzyingly complex and has enough intellectual fodder for lifetimes, but it is the moment-to-moment lived experience, unfiltered by figuring things out, that conveys presence. Similarly, as a physician with a long clinical, teaching, and research career, my "roses" are my connections with patients and colleagues. The work we do is often intellectually, physically, and emotionally difficult, and, as Montori and Heath point out, in medicine we need what the American

---

1   Heath, I., & Montori, V. M. (2023). Responding to the crisis of care. *BMJ Clinical Research*, *380*, 464. https://doi.org/10.1136/bmj.p464

suffragettes demanded in the early 20th century: "bread and roses." My development as a physician has been shaped as much by the sharing of presence, harmony, and communion with other human beings as it has through the "bread" of clinical practice—amassing and organizing facts, and diagnosing and solving problems.

In addition to knowledge and judgment, markers of an excellent clinician include attentiveness, curiosity, engagement, authenticity, and presence. I am not always sure what clinical wisdom is, but these must be some of the essential ingredients. As Shmuel Reis, Adina Kalet, and Wayne Weston emphasize in this book, insight and wisdom are not enough; to make a difference, these must be enacted in key moments of our clinical work. And the dark side—what gets doctors in trouble—rarely has to do with lack of knowledge, sometimes has to do with deficiencies in technical skill, but most often involves lack of self-awareness of one's own strengths and limitations and lack of an internal ethical compass. These, in turn, manifest as overconcreteness, unacknowledged negative emotions, inability to tolerate uncertainty, conflating wisdom with arrogance, and poor communication with patients and colleagues.

Our job as physicians is both transactional and interactional. The transactional is about acquisition and exchange, money for bread. Taking this to the extreme, the medical enterprise becomes an Orwellian factory, within which interchangeable workers submit to standardized quality control—an assemblage of competencies and entrustable professional activities. In this book, Drs. Reis, Kalet, and Weston, all experienced clinician-educators, argue that the transactional view is not enough. The interactional, they submit, is about growth and formation. This formative activity is more like planting a garden than running a factory.[2] One cannot force a professional to develop an identity, just as one cannot make a plant grow. Also, it is narrow to just talk about individual growth and formation. Our job as clinicians, educators, coaches, evaluators, and licensors is to provide an environment in which people can grow. This environment must provide essential nutrients. For roses, the ingredients are water, minerals, and sunlight. For physicians, the ingredients include psychological safety, community, agency, mentoring, and access to information. Similarly, the environment must afford protection. Roses need protection from extreme temperatures and wind. Clinicians need protection from cognitive, physical and emotional overload, injustice, and

2   Epstein, R. M. (2022). Mechanics and gardeners: The role of mindfulness in medical education. *Clinical Teacher*, 19(S1), 8–10. https://doi.org/10.1111/tct.13495

abuse. In too many current medical settings, nutrients and protection often are lacking.

When considering the models of professional development so comprehensively presented in this book, I am left with questions. First, *development towards what?* Some *whats* are enduring and universal, whereas others are highly contextual. You might say, *health*. Interestingly, though, there is no commonly accepted definition of health, at least in the USA.[3] Government agencies—the National Institutes of Health, the Health Resources and Services Administration, and the Centers for Medicare & Medicaid Services—do not have one. Similarly, consensual agreement about what makes a good doctor is lacking. Some time ago, Ed Hundert and I made an attempt at a definition of professional competence: "the habitual and judicious use of communication, knowledge, technical skills, clinical reasoning, emotions, values, and reflection in daily practice for the benefit of the individual and the community being served."[4] We continued by arguing that professional competence depends as much on the synthesis of these attributes as on their individual qualities.

Three years earlier, I wrote about the qualities of mind of exemplary physicians and, in a *JAMA* publication, described "mindful practice" as moment-to-moment purposeful attentiveness to one's own physical and mental processes during everyday work with the goal of practicing with clarity, competence, wisdom, and compassion.[5] By extension, efforts toward professional development or identity formation should nourish self-actualization, health-promoting behaviors, and communities of practice. What I missed 20 years ago were the threats to the sustainability of the healthcare workforce. Currently, a frightening number of physicians are leaving practice and retiring early. This trend involves much more than a lack of professional development or identity formation. Rather, in the USA and elsewhere, it reflects an environment that is excessively transactional and insufficiently interactional. The administrative technology of coding and billing is not balanced by the human technology of growth, flourishing, and awareness.

Those enacting models of professional development and identity formation need to know how to set the bar. Assessing medical knowledge is

---

3   Fiscella, K., & Epstein, R. M. (2023). The profound implications of the meaning of health for health care and health equity. *Milbank Quarterly*, *101*(3), 675–699. https://doi.org/10.1111/1468-0009.12660

4   Epstein, R. M., & Hundert, E. M. (2002). Defining and assessing professional competence. *JAMA*, *287*(2), 226–235. https://doi.org/10.1001/jama.287.2.226

5   Epstein, R. M. (1999). Mindful practice. *JAMA*, *282*(9), 833–839. https://doi.org/10.1001/jama.282.9.833

complex but more straightforward than assessing wisdom. None of us is superhuman, however much we are encouraged to act as if we might be. *Assuming that empathy and communication skills are essential to clinical practice, how does the manifestation (and assessment) of these skills differ in academic pathology and rural primary care settings? How is embodiment different for a surgeon and a psychiatrist?* Generalizations from moral philosophy and developmental psychology must be subjected to the realities of pragmatic engagement. In his book *Pragmatism*, William James describes philosophies as context-dependent, that no ideal applies to all situations.[6] Often we stumble along until we find the right match between theory and action.

I have never felt that I "fit in" to the prevailing culture of medicine or medical training. Coming to medicine after studying music and philosophy, and even after having had a rich and rewarding career as a clinician, teacher, and researcher, too often I have found the culture of medicine to be intellectually stultifying, emotionally silencing, socially unjust, and physically exhausting. I am not alone; many of my colleagues don't feel that they fit in either. I was fortunate, though, to have found enough shining lights to keep me going and growing. These mentors and colleagues, by example, demonstrated how one could be a full human being with an authentic, creative, unique, and caring identity that could make a difference. Sometimes formative moments occurred in very brief contacts with teachers and colleagues with insight, integrity, and presence. In addition, most of these shining lights engaged in quiet rebellions, questioning and refusing to submit to rigid definitions of physicianhood. Perhaps, then, part of the work of professional development and identity formation has a paradoxical quality to it, encouraging sufficient civil disobedience, anarchy, and subversiveness to follow one's inner compass while at the same time enacting our collective need to create and participate in communities of care, learning, inquiry, and practice.

While medical schools have made important progress in recognizing the importance of—and assessing—efforts to improve professional development and identity formation, once physicians complete formal training, professional development is piecemeal and chaotic. This book is an important step in providing a philosophical and moral framework for developing those to whom all of us will entrust our lives. The next steps will require ongoing insight into and expertise in vitalizing the multiple biopsychosocial levels that inform the human development of

---

6   James, W. (1975). *Pragmatism.* Harvard University Press.

physicians. Those insights will require collaboration among those with expertise in the neurocognitive, philosophical, narrative, moral/ethical, educational, psychological, and embodied dimensions of doctoring, as well as those with political, financial, and organizational expertise to enact programs that will make a difference. Importantly, we should be aware of the perils of getting lost in an attempt to "get it right." We will need to invoke the "science of muddling through,"[7] moving forward incrementally, with a moral compass but without knowing which of many paths we need to take, and recognizing that our understanding of professional development is continually evolving.

---

7   Lindblom, C. E. (1959). The science of "muddling through." *Public Administration Review*, *19*(2), 79–88. https://doi.org/10.2307/973677

Appendix

LITERATURE SEARCH STRATEGY (MEDICAL SUBJECT HEADINGS [MeSH])

General search terms: Physician or doctor life cycle or lifespan; Professional identity formation; Becoming a physician or doctor; Personal and professional development and physician or doctor; Professionalism and medicine and development; Developmental stages and growth of physicians; Identity development in medicine; Becoming a physician.

Specific search terms: Expertise in medicine; CME; Narrative medicine; Reflective practice; Moral development; Moral reasoning; Moral distress; Moral injury; Character development.

Index

For Product Safety Concerns and Information please contact our EU
representative GPSR@taylorandfrancis.com
Taylor & Francis Verlag GmbH, Kaufingerstraße 24, 80331 München, Germany